LANGE

USMLE ROAD MAP

FAMILY MEDICINE

PAUL GORDON, MD, MPH

Associate Professor
Family and Community Medicine
College of Medicine
The University of Arizona
Tucson, Arizona

Mc Graw Hill

New York Chicago San Francisco Lisbon London Madrid Mexico City
Milan New Delhi San Juan Seoul Singapore Sydney Toronto

The McGraw-Hill Companies

USMLE Road Map: Family Medicine, First Edition

1234567890 DOC/DOC 09876

ISBN-13: 978-0-07-146543-4

ISBN-10: 0-07-146543-X

Notice

Medicine is an ever-changing science. As new research and clinical experience broaden our knowledge, changes in treatment and drug therapy are required. The authors and the publisher of this work have checked with sources believed to be reliable in their efforts to provide information that is complete and generally in accord with the standards accepted at the time of publication. However, in view of the possibility of human error or changes in medical sciences, neither the authors nor the publisher nor any other party who has been involved in the preparation or publication of this work warrants that the information contained herein is in every respect accurate or complete, and they disclaim all responsibility for any errors or omissions or for the results obtained from use of the information contained in this work. Readers are encouraged to confirm the information contained herein with other sources. For example and in particular, readers are advised to check the product information sheet included in the package of each drug they plan to administer to be certain that the information contained in this work is accurate and that changes have not been made in the recommended dose or in the contraindications for administration. This recommendation is of particular importance in connection with new or infrequently used drugs.

This book was set in Adobe Garamond by Pine Tree Composition, Inc.
The editors were Jason Malley, Karen Edmonson, and Mary E. Bele.
The production supervisor was Catherine H. Saggese.
The index was prepared by Andover Publishing Services.

RR Donnelley was printer and binder.

This book is printed on acid-free paper

Cataloging-in-Publication data for this title are on file with the Library of Congress.

INTERNATIONAL EDITION ISBN13: 978-0-07-110488-3 ISBN-10: 0-07-110488-7

CONTENTS

USING THE
USMLE ROAD MAP SERIES
FOR SUCCESSFUL REVIEW

What Is the Road Map Series?

Short of having your own personal tutor, the USMLE Road Map Series is the best source for efficient review of major concepts and information in the medical sciences.

Why Do You Need A Road Map?

It allows you to navigate quickly and easily through your pharmacology course notes and textbook and prepares you for USMLE and course examinations.

How Does the Road Map Series Work?

Outline Form: Connects the facts in a conceptual framework so that you understand the ideas and retain the information.

Color and Boldface: Highlights words and phrases that trigger quick retrieval of concepts and facts.

Clear Explanations: Are fine-tuned by years of student interaction. The material is written by authors selected for their excellence in teaching and their experience in preparing students for board examinations.

Illustrations: Provide the vivid impressions that facilitate comprehension and recall.

To my daughter, Miriam Gordon, for her enormous contribution to this book. She helped with the process of reviewing background literature and writing.

CHAPTER 1
ABDOMINAL PAIN

I. Defining Features

A. Pain or **discomfort in the upper abdomen** may be associated with abdominal fullness, early satiety, burning, belching, nausea, retching, or vomiting.

B. Patients with **dyspepsia** often have heartburn.

II. Epidemiology

A. **Dyspepsia occurs in 25% of the adult population** and accounts for 3% of general medical office visits.

B. It is the chief complaint of approximately 5–10% of patients presenting to an emergency department.

C. It is one of the top 10 ambulatory complaints.

III. Pathophysiology

A. Food or Drug Intolerance

1. **Food intolerance** is often acute and self-limited. It may be caused by eating too quickly, eating foods high in fat, eating during stressful situations, or drinking alcohol or coffee in excess.
2. **Intolerance to drugs,** including aspirin, nonsteroidal anti-inflammatory drugs (NSAIDs), antibiotics (metronidazole and macrolides), corticosteroids, iron preparations, and narcotics may cause dyspepsia.

B. Luminal Gastrointestinal (GI) Tract Dysfunction

1. About 15–20% of patients with dyspepsia have peptic ulcer disease (PUD).
2. Up to **20% of patients with dyspepsia have gastroesophageal reflux disease (GERD),** which may not accompany significant heartburn.
3. Gastric cancer is rare and present in 1% of patients with dyspepsia.
4. Other causes include gastroparesis (particularly in patients who have diabetes), lactose intolerance or malabsorption, and parasitic infections.

C. Helicobacter pylori Infection

1. There is a **20–50% prevalence of *H pylori*-associated chronic gastritis in patients with dyspepsia,** the same percentage as occurs in the general population.
2. Eradication of *H pylori* rarely eliminates dyspepsia.

D. Pancreatic Disease

1. **Chronic pancreatitis** is characterized by persistent inflammation of the pancreas. It causes attacks of abdominal pain and nausea and vomiting that are worsened by eating or drinking, especially alcohol.
2. **Pancreatic carcinoma** is a malignant tumor of the pancreas. Early stage pancreatic cancer usually does not cause symptoms and remains silent until the tumor blocks the common bile duct, resulting in abdominal pain and jaundice.

E. Biliary Tract Disease

1. **Gallstones,** whose predominant chemical composition is cholesterol or calcium bilirubinate, cause biliary tract disease.
2. Although biliary tract disease is a cause of dyspepsia, the acute onset and right upper quadrant character of cholelithiasis and choledocholithiasis should allow these conditions to be readily distinguished from dyspepsia.

F. Other Associated Medical Conditions Causing Abdominal Pain

1. Diabetes
2. Renal insufficiency
3. Thyroid disease
4. Myocardial ischemia
5. Intra-abdominal tumor
6. Volvulus
7. Pregnancy

G. Functional (Nonulcer) Dyspepsia

1. Functional, or nonulcer, dyspepsia is the **most common cause of chronic dyspepsia.**
2. Up to two thirds of patients have no obvious organic cause for their symptoms.
3. Symptoms are thought to arise from a complex interaction of increased afferent sensitivity, gastric-delayed emptying, and impaired accommodation to food or psychosocial stressors.
4. Although benign, symptoms may be chronic and difficult to treat.

IV. Risk Factors

A. Patients with **PUD** are usually **younger than 45** years, are **smokers,** and experience pain that is relieved by food or antacids.

B. Patients with nonulcer dyspepsia are younger, report a variety of abdominal and extra-abdominal complaints, show signs of anxiety or depression, or have a history of use of psychotropic medication.

V. Clinical Presentation

A. The **history** is one of the most important components and can help direct the remainder of the work-up.

1. **Chronic or acute pain:** Sudden onset of abdominal pain associated with hemodynamic changes requires emergent evaluation and intervention.
   a. **Pain that is severe and of sudden onset** often points to
      (1) Appendicitis
      (2) Leaking or ruptured abdominal aortic aneurysm (AAA)
      (3) Perforated ulcer

(4) Pancreatitis
(5) Obstruction (small or large bowel)
(6) Non-gastrointestinal sources, such as ectopic pregnancy, acute myocardial infarction (MI), or renal calculi

b. **Pain that is more chronic with gradual onset** may be caused by
(1) Functional bowel disease
(2) Celiac disease
(3) Constipation
(4) Chronic diarrhea
(5) GERD
(6) Non-gastrointestinal sources such as prostatitis, ovarian cysts, or pelvic inflammatory disease (PID)

2. **Quality of the pain** can help differentiate the etiology.
   a. **Burning pain** is often GERD.
   b. **Hunger-like sensation** is often seen in patients who have PUD.
   c. **"An elephant sitting on my chest"** often describes cardiac ischemia.
3. **Location and radiation of the pain** can be helpful in determining the diagnosis.
   a. **Periumbilical to right lower quadrant (RLQ) pain** often suggests acute appendicitis.
   b. **Mid-epigastric pain radiating to the back** suggests pancreatitis.
   c. **RUQ pain radiating to the scapula** suggests gallbladder disease.
4. **Pattern and frequency of the pain** can also be helpful in determining the diagnosis.
   a. If the **pain worsens when lying down and occurs after meals,** the diagnosis may be GERD.
   b. If **the pain occurs after consumption of a high-fat meal,** gallbladder disease is likely.
   c. If the **pain is relieved after a bowel movement,** consider functional abdominal pain.
5. **Other Signs and Symptoms Associated with Dyspepsia**
   a. Patients who have infections will often have **fever and chills.**
   b. Patients who have pancreatitis experience **nausea and vomiting.**
   c. If **hematemesis** is present, the diagnosis is PUD or a Mallory-Weiss tear.
   d. **Emotional stress** can exacerbate symptoms if they are due to functional abdominal disease.
   e. If **blood or melena** is present, this dictates the need for intraluminal investigation of the GI tract.

B. The **physical examination** must be thorough.
1. **Inspection:** Look for distention, scars, and striae.
   a. **Distention** suggests ascites or obstruction.
   b. **Scars** may be a sign of previous surgery and could lead to bowel obstruction.
   c. **Striae** suggest rapid abdominal growth.
2. **Auscultation**
   a. **Hypo- and hyperactive bowel sounds** can indicate a bowel obstruction, either partial or complete.
   b. **Bruits** over the aorta and renal and femoral arteries suggest aneurysm.
3. **Palpation**
   a. **Rebound tenderness with RLQ pain** suggests appendicitis.

b. **RUQ pain with inspiration** suggests acute cholecystitis.
c. **Rebound tenderness** indicates peritoneal irritation often related to a perforated viscus.

4. **Red flag findings:** The following findings are suggestive of serious organic disease and warrant further investigation (Table 1–1).
   a. Weight loss
   b. Organomegaly
   c. Abdominal mass
   d. Fecal occult blood

CLINICAL SKILLS TIP

If you suspect malingering, true rebound tenderness can be assessed by pounding the patient's heels. You can also ask the patient to hop off the table.

Table 1–1. Alarm features of dyspepsia.

Symptom	Consider this Diagnosis	Work-up
> 45 years (new onset)		
Rectal bleeding or melena	Peptic ulcer or colonic lesion	Endoscopy
Weight loss of ≥ 10% of body weight	Gastric carcinoma	Endoscopy
Anorexia/early satiety	Gastric carcinoma	Endoscopy
Persistent vomiting	PUD, brain malignancy	Endoscopy and CT scan of head
Anemia or bleeding	PUD, gastric carcinoma	Endoscopy
Progressive dysphagia or odynophagia	Esophageal or gastric carcinoma (Barrett's)	Endoscopy
Jaundice	Liver disease	Abdominal ultrasound or CT scan
Abdominal mass or lymphadenopathy	Neoplasm or lymphoma	Abdominal CT scan
Family history of cancer of the upper GI tract	Gastric carcinoma	Endoscopy
Previous gastric surgery or neoplasm	GI obstruction or malignancy	Kidneys, ureter, and bladder x-ray; endoscopy
Previous history of PUD	Gastric malignancy	Endoscopy

CT, computer tomography; GI, gastrointestinal; PUD, peptic ulcer disease.

VI. Differential Diagnosis

A. The differential diagnosis of abdominal pain is extensive and can be organized on an **organ-based** approach (see III).

B. Table 1–1 can be used to differentiate the worrisome or important rule-out causes of dyspepsia.

C. Figure 1–1 can be used to aid in differential diagnosis of abdominal pain.

RULE OUT

Although uncommon, it is important to rule out abdominal aortic aneurysm and intestinal ischemia or MI.

VII. Diagnostic Findings

A. **Upper endoscopy** is the study of choice to determine if gastroduodenal ulcers, erosive esophagitis, or neoplasms of the upper GI tract are present. Barium radiography is inferior to endoscopy.

B. An initial **noninvasive test for *H pylori*** (IgG serology, fecal antigen test, or urea breath test) should be performed in most young, uncomplicated patients with dyspepsia.

C. **Abdominal imaging studies,** including ultrasonography or computerized tomography (CT), should be performed when biliary tract disease or pancreatic disease is suspected.

D. **Gastric emptying studies** are valuable in patients who have recurrent vomiting.

E. **Ambulatory esophageal pH testing** is helpful in the diagnosis of patients who have atypical GERD.

VIII. Treatment (Figure 1–2)

A. There are **3 categories of pharmacologic agents** that enhance the healing of peptic ulcers.

1. **Acid antisecretory agents**
   a. **Proton pump inhibitors (PPIs)** inhibit 90% of 24-hour acid secretion when compared with 65% for H_2-receptor antagonists given in standard dosages. PPIs are remarkably safe when used as short-term therapy.
   b. **H_2-receptor antagonists** are effective in the treatment of PUD. Duodenal and gastric ulcer healing rates of 85–90% are obtained with 6 and 8 weeks of therapy, respectively.
2. **Mucosal protective agents** such as sucralfate, bismuth, misoprostol, and low doses of aluminum-containing antacids have been shown to promote ulcer healing. They are rarely used now because of the greater efficacy and ease of use of PPIs and H_2-receptor antagonists.
3. **Agents that promote healing through eradication of *H pylori*** are now used as the gold standard in the treatment of ulcer disease. Eradication has proved difficult and requires multiple agents. Multiple regimens are available and generally include two antibiotics and a PPI. All regimens achieve eradication rates of > 85% after 10–14 days of treatment (Table 1–2).

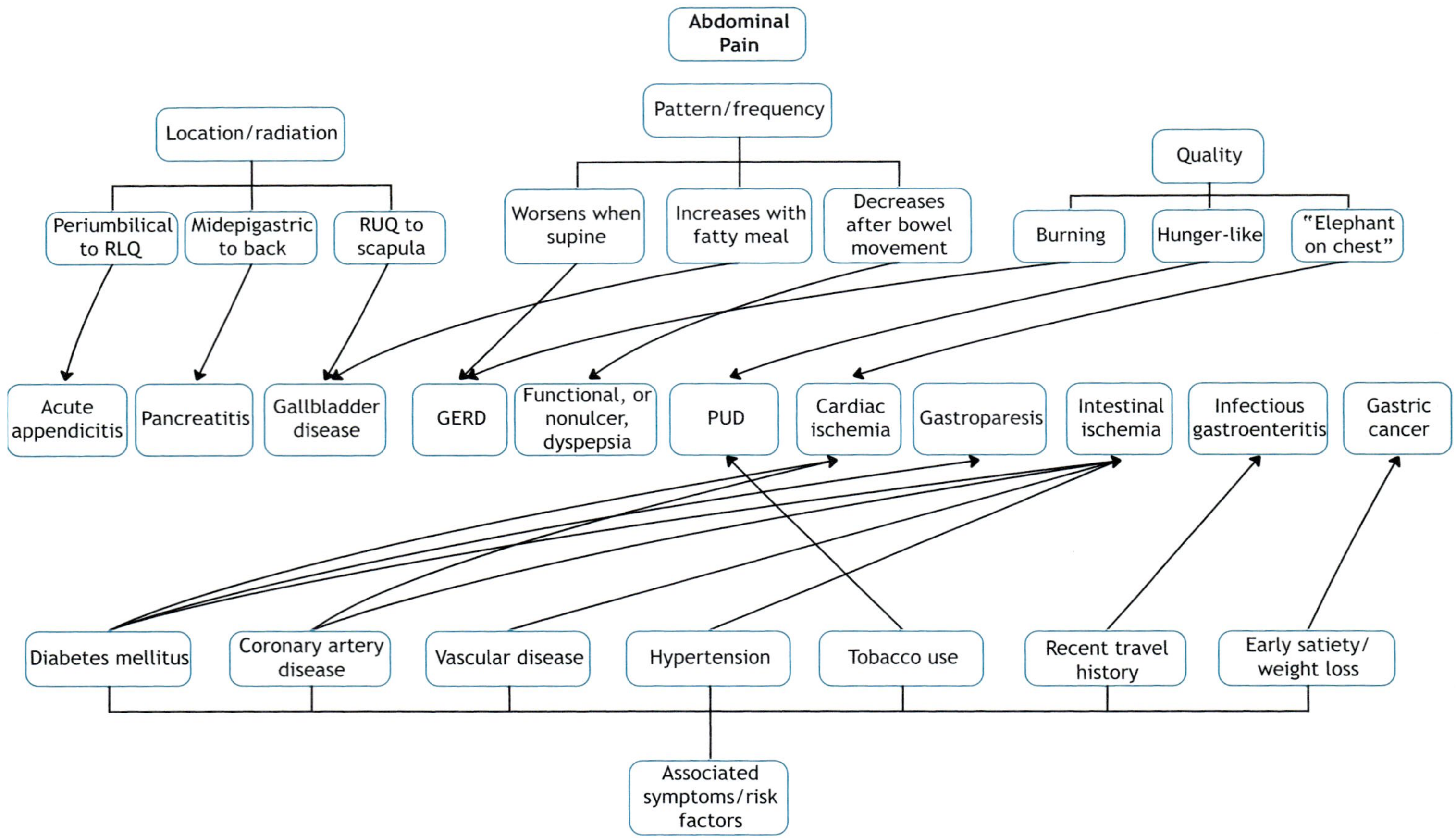

Figure 1–1. Differential diagnosis of abdominal pain.

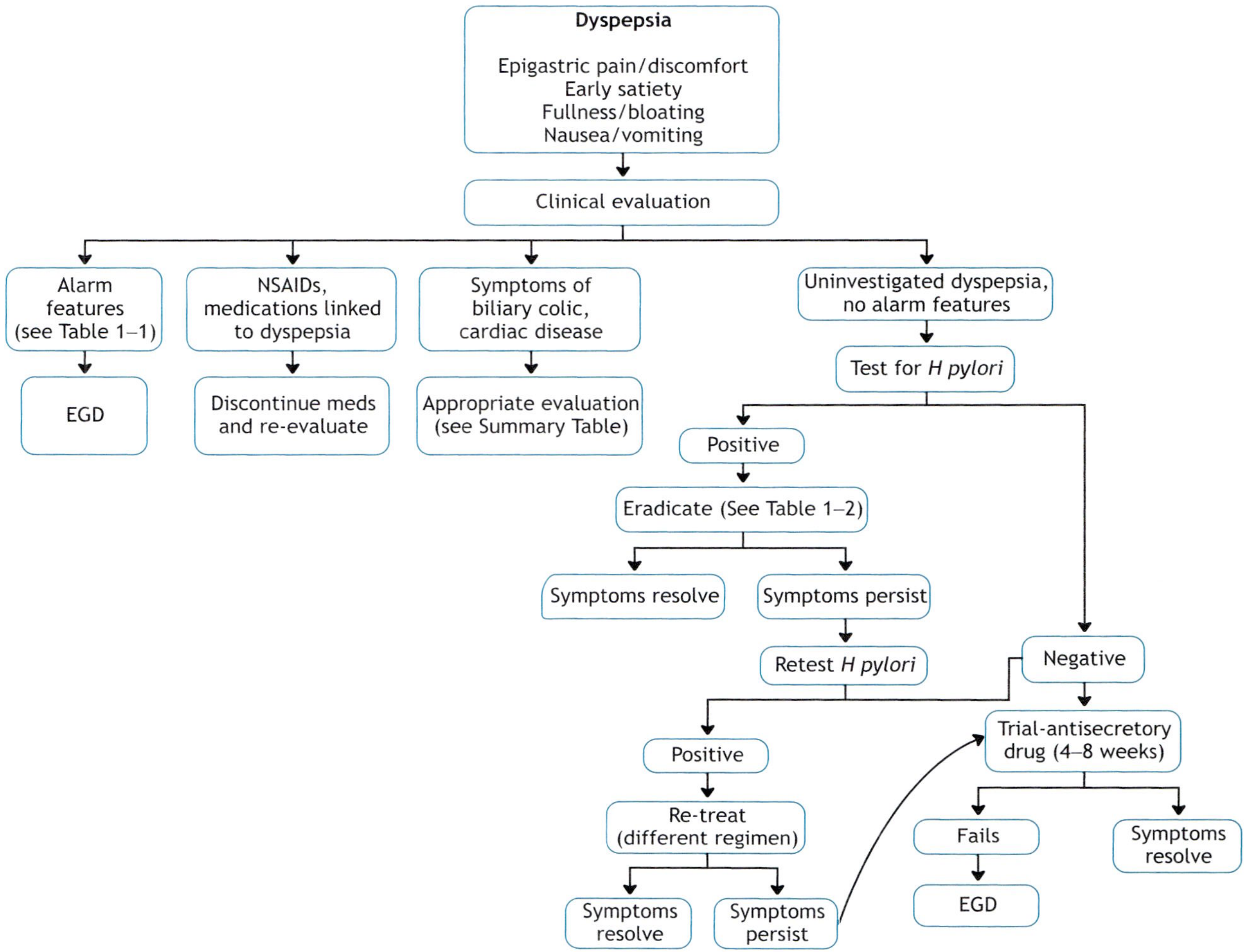

Figure 1–2. Treatment algorithm for dyspepsia.

Table 1–2. Treatment options for *H pylori* infection.

Treat with anti-*H pylori* regimen for 10–14 days:
• PPI 2 times a day (omeprazole 20 mg, rabeprazole 20 mg, lansoprazole 30 mg, or pantoprazole 40 mg; esomeprazole 40 mg (give only once a day) • Clarithromycin 500 mg 2 times a day • Amoxicillin 1 gm 2 times a day (or metronidazole 500 mg 2 times a day if allergic to penicillin)
• PPI 2 times a day • Bismuth subsalicylate 2 tablets 4 times a day • Tetracycline 500 mg 4 times a day • Metronidazole 250 mg 4 times a day
• Ranitidine bismuth citrate 400 mg 2 times a day (not available in USA) • Clarithromycin 500 mg 2 times a day • Amoxicillin 1gm or tetracycline 500 mg (or metronidazole 500 mg 2 times a day if allergic to penicillin)
After completion of 10–14 day course of therapy to eradicate *H pylori*, continue treatment with PPI or H_2-receptor antagonist for 4-8 weeks to promote healing.

PPI, proton pump inhibitor.

B. **Treatment of functional or nonulcer dyspepsia** presents a separate challenge and can be divided into 4 categories.

1. **General Measures**
   a. A **stable physician-patient relationship is critically important.** Patients require reassurance in knowing that their condition is not serious but that it may be chronic.
   b. Alcohol **and caffeine consumption should be reduced or eliminated.** Keeping a diary of symptoms may help the patient identify a psychological precipitant of their pain.
2. **Pharmacologic Agents**
   a. **Antisecretory therapy** with either an H_2-receptor antagonist or a PPI for 2–4 weeks will benefit 10–30% of patients (one third of patients benefit from placebo).
   b. Low doses of **antidepressants** may benefit some patients through moderation of visceral afferent sensitivity. Side-effects, however, are common.
   c. Prokinetic agents are unlikely to lead to significant improvement; metoclopramide has a high incidence of neuropsychiatric side-effects with long-term use.
3. **Anti-*H pylori* treatment:** 5–15% of patients may derive benefit from eradication of *H pylori*.
4. **Alternative therapies:** Psychotherapy and hypnotherapy may benefit selected motivated patients. Herbal therapies such as peppermint and caraway may offer some benefit with minimal risk.

IX. Summary Table

Disease	Pathophysiology	Diagnostic Studies	Treatment
PUD	Excess acid	EGD; *H pylori*	Anti-*H pylori* regimen; +/- antisecretory drugs
GERD	Reflux of gastric acid	EGD; *H pylori*	Antisecretory drugs and prokinetic agents; anti-*H pylori* regimen if positive
Gastroparesis	Autonomic dysfunction	FBS; gastric emptying study	Prokinetic agents
Lactose intolerance	Lactase deficiency	None	Lactase enzyme supplementation
Infectious gastroenteritis	Luminal infection	Cultures; stool for leukocytes	Appropriate antibiotics
NSAID or other drug-related condition	Drug effect on GI lumen	None	Stop medication
Gastric cancer	Neoplasm in GI tract	EGD	As directed by type of tumor
H pylori-associated chronic gastritis	Infectious disease	*H pylori* serology, fecal antigen test or urea breath test	Anti-*H pylori* regimen
Pancreatitis	Inflammatory destruction of pancreatic cells	Lipase, amylase; possibly ERCP	Hospitalization, bowel rest, analgesia
Biliary tract disease	Inflammatory or obstructive (stone-related)	Abdominal ultrasound and/or CT scan and/or ERCP	Antibiotics as appropriate; consideration for surgery
Functional (nonulcer) dyspepsia	Possibly from interaction of increased afferent sensitivity, gastric-delayed emptying, and impaired accommodation to food	None	Good physician-patient relationship; anti-*H pylori* regimen; and/or alternative therapies including psychotherapy and hypnotherapy

DM, diabetes mellitus; EGD, esophagastroduodenoscopy; ERCP, endoscopic retrograde cholangiopancreatography; FBS, fasting blood sugar; GI, gastrointestinal; NSAID, nonsteroidal anti-inflammatory drug.

CLINICAL CASE

A 44-year-old man presents with a 1-year history of intermittent pain in the epigastric region. The pain often occurs 1 hour after a meal. The pain does not radiate, and the patient has not experienced weight loss, vomiting, or symptoms of gastrointestinal bleeding. He denies early satiety, bloating, constipation, or diarrhea. He reports heartburn about 2 times a month, typically when he goes to bed soon after eating a large meal. He is otherwise healthy, is not obese, and takes no medications.

This is a common presentation to the office of a primary care physician. The patient has a bothersome symptom but no alarm features. As shown in Figure 1–1, he should be tested for H pylori. *If the test is positive, he should be treated with an appropriate regimen. If the test is negative, he should be given a trial of an antisecretory drug for 4–8 weeks. If all investigations and therapies fail to alleviate this patient's symptoms, a diagnosis of nonulcer (functional) dyspepsia can be made. The treatments outlined in Table 1–2 may benefit him, but it is important that he understand that his condition, although not serious, may be chronic. Patients with this diagnosis should also be advised that treatment of the infection may or may not alleviate their symptoms in the short term and may even aggravate them. Clinical trials have shown that eradication of* H pylori *infection relieves symptoms of nonulcer dyspepsia in a small group of infected individuals. Treatment can be offered on the basis that 1 in 15 infected persons may have symptomatic improvement.*

Serologic testing for H pylori *infection relies on detection of IgG antibodies to* H pylori. *Serology tests performed in the office of the primary care physician have not reached acceptable accuracy for the diagnosis of* H pylori *infection. The urea breath test (UBT) is a reliable test performed both before and after treatment and is the test of choice for determining cure of infection when clinically indicated and when repeat endoscopy is not necessary. Serology is an inappropriate means of detecting cure of infection; the test of choice is the endoscopic testing biopsy urease test. Culture is an impractical means of diagnosing* H pylori *infection.*

If our patient were older than age 45 and presented with hematochezia or melena; experienced a new onset of symptoms and had early satiety, anorexia, or a weight loss of 10% of his body weight; or experienced any of the alarm features listed in Table 1–1, an endoscopy should be performed immediately. Similarly, if his symptoms were drug-related (eg, NSAIDs, narcotics), you should recommend discontinuing the medications and re-evaluating him within 4 weeks. Symptoms suggestive of biliary tract disease should lead you to investigate performing ultrasound or CT scan of the RUQ.

H pylori *infection predisposes to both the intestinal and diffuse types of gastric cancer; however, there are no known predictors for the development of gastric cancer in infected individuals. It is recommended that patients who have* H pylori *infection be treated following surgery for early gastric cancer. Screening asymptomatic individuals for* H pylori *infection as a means of reducing the incidence of gastric cancer currently is not recommended.*

CLINICAL PEARLS

H pylori *is a common organism that can cause gastrointestinal disease. Treatment is important.*

CHAPTER 2
ANXIETY

I. Defining Features

A. Anxiety is an **overt manifestation of a defense mechanism or a phobia,** or both.

B. **Somatic symptoms** are referable to the **autonomic nervous system** or to a **specific organ system** (eg, dyspnea, palpitations, paresthesias).

C. **Most laboratory studies are normal in patients with anxiety disorders.**

D. The *Diagnostic and Statistical Manual of Mental Disorders,* 4th edition, text revision (DSM-IV-TR), recognizes the following **subtypes of anxiety disorders** (Table 2–1):

1. **Acute stress disorder:** Person has been exposed to a traumatic event in which both of the following were present:
   a. The person experienced, witnessed, or was confronted with an event or events that involved actual or threatened death or serious injury or a threat to the physical integrity of self or others.
   b. The person's response involved intense fear, helplessness, or horror.
2. **Panic disorder with agoraphobia:** Recurrent unexpected attacks with at least 1 attack associated with concern about additional attacks, worries about the implications of the attack, or a significant change in behavior related to the attack leads to agoraphobia.
3. **Generalized anxiety disorder (GAD):** Persistent underlying anxiety and significant symptoms of motor tension, autonomic hyperactivity, and hypervigilance lasting more than 6 months.
4. **Obsessive compulsive disorder (OCD):** Persistent unwanted and disturbing thoughts and recurrent behavioral patterns (eg, hand washing) that interfere with daily life.
5. **Panic disorder without agoraphobia:** Unprovoked panic attacks.
6. **Post-traumatic stress disorder (PTSD):** Recurrent flashbacks or nightmares by survivors of a catastrophic event; often associated with panic attacks and major depression.
7. **Adjustment disorder with anxiety:** Developmentally inappropriate and excessive anxiety concerning separation from home or from those to whom the individual is attached.
8. **Social phobia (social anxiety disorder):** Marked and persistent fear and avoidance of performance or social situations in which the person is exposed to unfamiliar people or scrutiny.

Table 2–1. DSM-IV-TR classification of anxiety disorders and their main symptoms.

Disorder	Symptom
Acute stress disorder	Trauma causing intense fear lasting < 1 month
Panic disorder with agoraphobia	Panic attacks with avoidance of situations where escape is difficult or embarrassing
GAD	Excessive worry about a number of events or activities on most days for at least 6 months
OCD	Repeated, intrusive thoughts or images or actions that are recognized as excessive
Panic disorder without agoraphobia	Recurrent unexpected panic attacks
PTSD	Trauma causing intense fear and reexperiencing of trauma lasting > 1 month
Adjustment disorder with anxiety	Stressor or life event temporally related to onset of anxiety symptoms
SAD/social phobia	Fear and avoidance of situations involving potential negative evaluation and scrutiny by others
Specific phobia	Persistent, unreasonable fear and avoidance of a feared object or situation

GAD, generalized anxiety disorder; OCD, obsessive compulsive disorder; PTSD, post-traumatic stress disorder; SAD, social anxiety disorder.

9. **Specific phobia:** Intense recurrent fear of, and avoidance of, an object or situation.

II. Epidemiology

A. About 40 million people in the United States have some type of anxiety disorder.

B. **Generalized anxiety disorder is the most common type of anxiety disorder.**

C. **Panic disorders affect 3–5% of the population** and usually begin **before age 25.**

D. **Women have a greater tendency than men to have panic attacks.**

E. About 2–3% of the population has obsessive compulsive disorder (OCD).

F. In **two thirds of patients with OCD,** there is an **onset of depression.**

III. Pathophysiology

A. Anxiety symptoms and the resulting disorders are thought to be due to **disrupted modulation within the central nervous system and a reinforcement of further anxiety.**

B. Anxiety can become self-generating because the symptoms reinforce the reaction, causing the reaction to spiral.

C. Anxiety is often an epiphenomenon of other medical or psychiatric disorders.

IV. Risk Factors

A. Social and financial problems

B. Medical illness

C. Family history

D. Lack of social support

V. Clinical Presentation

A. Symptoms of Anxiety Disorders

1. Unrealistic or excessive anxiety or worry
2. Sense of impending doom
3. Nervousness
4. Palpitations
5. Hyperventilation with choking sensation
6. Nausea or abdominal distress
7. Paresthesias
8. Diaphoresis
9. Dizziness or syncope
10. Chest tightness and pressure (pseudoangina)

B. Signs of Anxiety Disorders

1. Tachycardia
2. Systolic click murmur
3. Labile hypertension
4. Sighing respiration
5. Muscle tension
6. Muscle spasm

CLINICAL SKILLS TIP

Although many signs and symptoms related to anxiety are common, it is important to consider other diagnoses.

VI. Differential Diagnosis

A. Cardiovascular

1. Ischemic heart disease
2. Valvular heart disease, including mitral valve prolapse (most symptomatic cases are associated with panic disorder)
3. Cardiomyopathies
4. Arrhythmias

B. Respiratory

1. Asthma
2. Emphysema
3. Pulmonary embolism

C. Central Nervous System
1. Transient cerebral insufficiency
2. Psychomotor epilepsy
3. Essential tremor

D. Metabolic and Hormonal
1. Hyperthyroidism
2. Pheochromocytoma
3. Adrenal insufficiency
4. Cushing syndrome
5. Hypokalemia, hypoglycemia
6. Hyperparathyroidism
7. Myasthenia gravis

E. Nutritional
1. Thiamine, pyridoxine, or folate deficiencies
2. Iron deficiency anemia

F. Intoxication
1. Excess caffeine
2. Alcohol
3. Cocaine
4. Sympathomimetics
5. Amphetamines

G. Withdrawal
1. Alcohol
2. Sedative-hypnotics

H. Other
1. Depression
2. Panic disorder associated with several physical disorders include
   a. Mitral valve prolapse (systolic click-murmur)
   b. Labile hypertension
   c. Migraine headaches
   d. Irritable bowel syndrome
   e. Asthma (chronic obstructive pulmonary disease, COPD)

RULE OUT

As well as the conditions listed above, the physician must ascertain if

- *The patient is at serious risk of committing suicide.*
- *The patient has psychotic symptoms.*
- *There are coexisting drug and/or alcohol problems.*

VII. Diagnostic Findings (Figure 2–1)

A. Laboratory Studies
1. Complete blood cell count (CBC) and urinalysis
2. Blood chemistries
3. Thyroid function studies

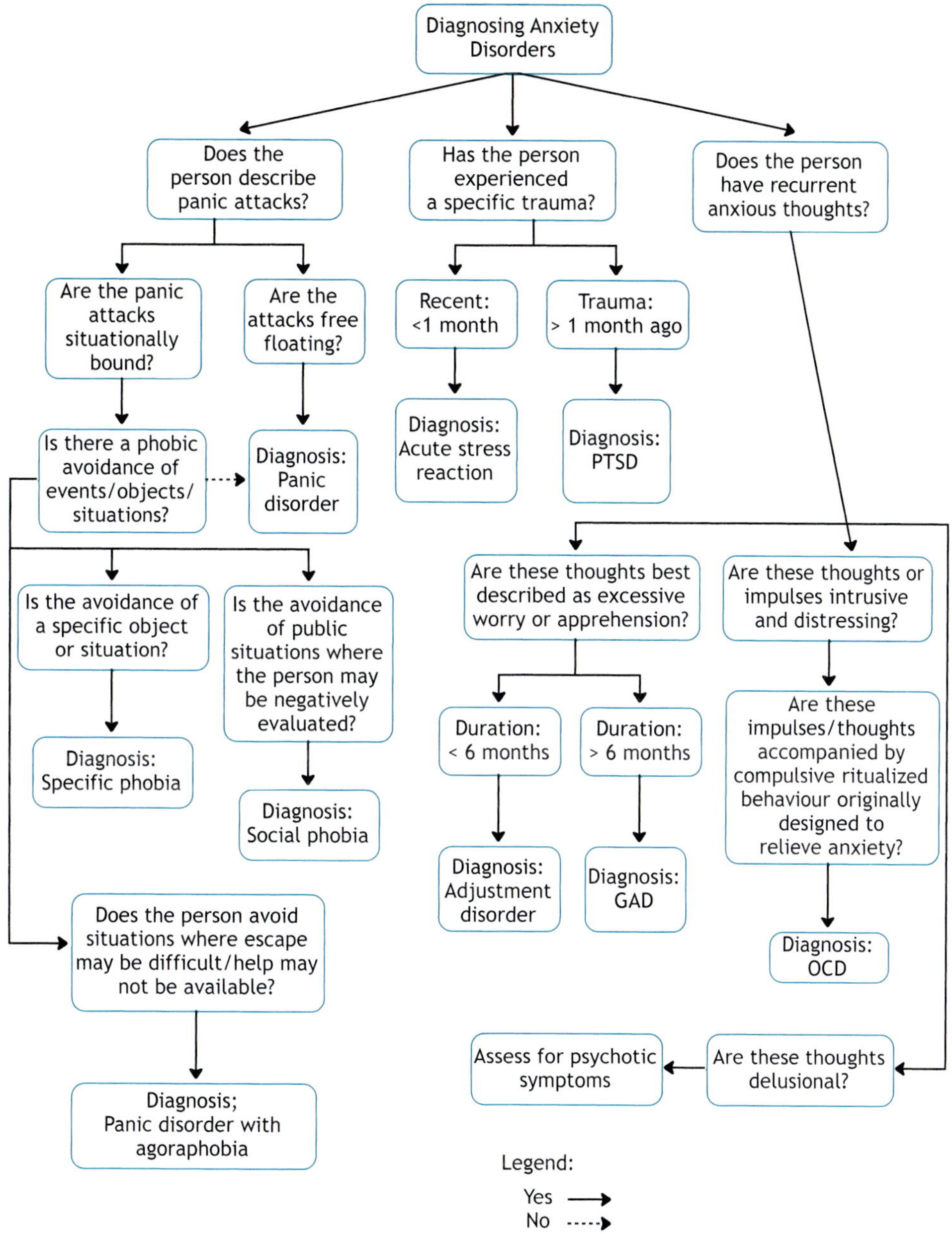

Figure 2–1 Diagnosing anxiety disorders.

B. Diagnostic Procedures

1. **Psychological testing** (eg, Spitzer's Patient Health Questionnaire, Hamilton's anxiety scale)
2. **Interview patient based on DSM-IV-TR** (see Clinical Case)

VIII. Treatment (Table 2–2)

A. Generalized Anxiety Disorder

1. **Benzodiazepines** are the most affective drug used in the acute management of GAD.
2. **Antidepressants,** including tricyclic antidepressants (**TCAs**) and selective serotonin reuptake inhibitors (**SSRIs**), can be helpful for long-term treatment.

Table 2–2. Summary of effective treatment strategies in anxiety disorders.

Disorder	Non-pharmacologic Therapy	Pharmacotherapy
Acute stress disorder	Cognitive behavioral therapy Psychological debriefing Anxiety management groups	Short term benzodiazepines (<4 weeks) SSRIs Clomipramine
Panic disorder with agoraphobia	Education about nature of disorder Behavioral therapy: controlled breathing, graded exposure to feared situations Group therapy Specialist referral to a cognitive behavioral program for nonresponders	SSRIs TCAs Benzodiazepines
GAD	Education about nature of disorder Support (guidance, advice) Counseling Relaxation therapy Stress management (relaxation, meditation) Behavioral therapy: structured problem solving, graded exposure to difficult situations Specialist referral to a cognitive behavioral program for nonresponders	SSRIs Venlafaxine TCAs Benzodiazepines β blockers
OCD	Education about nature of disorder Behavior therapy (ie, training in exposure to the provoking stimuli) Cognitive therapy: patient taught to challenge the validity of his fears and to resist carrying out compulsions Specialist referral to a cognitive behavioral therapy program recommended	SSRIs Clomipramine

(continued)

Table 2–2. Summary of effective treatment strategies in anxiety disorders. (*continued*)

Disorder	Non-pharmacologic Therapy	Pharmacotherapy
Panic disorder without agoraphobia	Education about nature of disorder Behavioral therapy: controlled breathing, graded exposure to feared situations Group therapy: groups of patients with similar problems directed by a trained therapist	SSRIs TCAs Benzodiazepines
PSTD	Psychoeducation Self-help and management Cognitive therapy Stress inoculation training Exposure in vivo to safe triggers of generalized avoidance Supportive counseling Treatment of comorbid disorders, especially depression Specialist referral to a cognitive behavioral program recommended	SSRIs TCAs Benzodiazepines
Adjustment disorder with anxiety	Individual psychotherapy Family therapy Behavior therapy Self-help support groups	Antianxiety medication (eg, lorazepam 1 mg 3 times a day, or clonazepam 0.5-1.5 mg at bedtime) < 2 weeks
SAD/social phobia	Behavior therapy (ie, exposure to the feared social situation)	SSRIs TCAs Benzodiazepines β blockers
Specific phobias	Behavior therapy (ie, exposure to the feared situation or object)	Drugs alone are generally not helpful

GAD, generalized anxiety disorder; OCD, obsessive compulsive disorder; PTSD, post-traumatic stress disorder; SAD, social anxiety disorder; SSRI, selective serotonin reuptake inhibitor; TCA, tricyclic antidepressant.

B. Panic Disorder

1. Sublingual dose of **lorazepam or alprazolam** is effective for urgent treatment during a panic attack.
2. **SSRIs** can be used for long-term treatment.
3. **High-potency benzodiazepines** can be used for short-term treatment.
4. **Clonazepam** (longer-acting) is an effective alternative to antidepressants.
5. **Antidepressants in conjunction with β blockers** can be used in resistant cases.

C. Phobia Disorders

1. Phobia disorders can be treated with the **same drugs that are used to treat panic attacks** (see Table 2–2).
2. Global social phobias may be treated with **SSRIs** (eg, paroxetine, sertraline, fluvoxamine) or with **monoamine oxidase inhibitors (MAOIs).**
3. Performance anxiety can be treated with **β blockers** (eg, propranolol).
4. **Serotonergic drugs** have proved to be 60% effective in patients who are diagnosed with **OCD.**
5. **Clomipramine** can be used to treat phobia disorders.

CLINICAL CASE

A 45-year-old woman sees her physician because she is worried that she has a brain tumor. She tells you that she has had a headache at least 2 times a week for the past 2 weeks. She further states that she has been diagnosed with tension headaches, but these headaches are different. One week ago, she was evaluated by her primary care practitioner, who told her she was having tension headaches and tried to tell her not to worry. She was not reassured and went to the emergency department (ED) 2 nights ago. While there, blood tests, a head CT scan, and a lumbar puncture were performed. The record from the ED confirms that the tests were normal. Nonetheless, the patient still thinks she has a brain tumor. On further questioning, you learn that she always worries about everything and has been called "the worrywart." This has been occurring for over 1 year. After further questioning, she denies any symptoms consistent with thyroid dysfunction. Review of her past medical history reveals tension headaches, 2 normal pregnancies, and multiple office visits for viral illnesses. She takes ibuprofen for her tension headaches and does well with it. She has had no surgeries. She is a single parent of 2 adolescent children. She has worked in the county recorder's office for the past 10 years. She does not use alcohol, tobacco, or illegal drugs. On physical examination, her vital signs are all normal. She appears anxious while sitting somewhat uncomfortably on the examination table and moving about more than most patients do. HEENT and funduscopic examinations are normal. Heart and lungs sounds are without abnormality. Her neurologic examination reveals a normal mental status and a non-focal examination.

This patient presents with an extremely common condition: anxiety. There are multiple types of anxiety disorders as well as other conditions that mimic anxiety symptoms. The physician's first task is to be certain that the other conditions are absent, which include disorders related to the following systems or categories (see VI):

1. Cardiovascular
2. Respiratory
3. Central nervous system
4. Metabolic and hormonal
5. Nutritional
6. Intoxication
7. Withdrawal

Fortunately for the physician, disorders related to these systems have a constellation of signs and symptoms that will facilitate a diagnosis. However, appropriate laboratory investigations and diagnostic studies may be necessary. **Basic screening tests** to identify some of these medical conditions may include

1. CBC
2. Serum chemistries
3. Thyroid-stimulating hormone (TSH)
4. Electrocardiogram (ECG)
5. Chest x-ray

Based on the specific signs and symptoms elicited from the patient, the physician will be better able to direct the diagnostic investigation.

Anxiety is an emotion experienced by everyone in daily life. It is a physical, emotional, and behavioral response to perceived threats. **Anxiety** can spur someone to better performance; however, it **can become a problem and is considered to be a disorder when**

1. It is of greater intensity and/or duration than would be expected in the given circumstances.
2. It affects daily life.
3. It gives rise to unexplained physical symptoms.
4. It leads to avoidance of situations and places.

Psychosocial assessment is an important aspect of the history of a patient in whom there is consideration of an anxiety disorder. This assessment should include

1. Nature of developmental factors
2. Life stressors and conflicts
3. Social support and resources
4. Current living situation
5. Financial concerns
6. Questions regarding domestic or relationship violence

Table 2–1 lists the types of anxiety disorders and their major symptoms. Figure 2–1 is an algorithm that the physician can use to help in the diagnosis of the specific type of anxiety disorder.

In the primary care setting, the physician must determine if a **referral to a psychiatrist** for consultation is appropriate. **The following factors suggest the need for referral.** When

1. There is a serious risk of suicide.
2. There are psychotic symptoms.
3. There are coexisting drug and/or alcohol problems.
4. Symptoms are severe or complex.
5. Symptoms fail to improve on initial treatment and follow-up.

Once the diagnosis is confirmed, the physician will focus on **treatment,** which may include **psychosocial intervention** (eg, psychological therapy and community-based support groups) and **pharmacotherapy.** Pharmacotherapy is indicated when

1. Symptoms are severe.
2. There is significant impairment of social, occupational, and role functioning.
3. There is concurrent moderate or severe depressive disorder.

Antidepressants are recommended as effective agents for **the treatment of panic disorders, social phobia, OCDs, GAD, and PTSD. SSRIs** are recommended as **first-line drug treatment for anxiety disorder.** The lowest effective dose of benzodiazepines to achieve symptom relief should be used over a limited period, and the dose should be gradually tapered off. Long-term use should be closely supervised for adverse effects, abuse, tolerance, dependency, and withdrawal symptoms.

Because **relapse is common** after discontinuation of medication for most anxiety disorders, **long-term maintenance treatment is recommended** following the amelioration of acute symptoms. Long-term maintenance therapy strongly predicts continued remission following discontinuation of medications. Medication for most patients with OCD should be continued for at least 1 year. After improvement with use of medication, antidepressant treatment for panic disorders and social phobias should be continued for at least 6 months.

A gradual taper of medication over a longer period (eg, 6 months) is recommended to prevent relapse. Relapse rates can be 90% with abrupt discontinuation of medication. Medication should be tapered off gradually, over a period of several weeks, titrating against symptoms to avoid withdrawal syndrome and symptom rebound. Longer-acting benzodiazepines are less likely to cause withdrawal and may be used during the tapering period to ameliorate symptoms. Discontinuation of antidepressants poses less of a problem in terms of withdrawal symptoms, although changes in mood, affect, appetite, and sleep may occur with SSRI discontinuation and more so with a shorter-acting SSRI such as paroxetine (see Table 2–2).

There is evidence that **continuation of psychological therapy sessions** during long-term follow-up can further **lead to improvement and reduce relapse.** Cognitive behavior therapy (CBT) may facilitate the tapering of benzodiazepines.

CLINICAL PEARLS

Anxiety is a common condition, and there are multiple types of anxiety disorders. Symptoms can mimic other medical conditions.

CHAPTER 3

ALLERGIC RHINITIS

I. Defining Features

A. **Seasonal or perennial occurrence** of nasal pruritus, congestion, rhinorrhea, or paroxysms of sneezing may be associated with lower respiratory tract symptoms, eye erythema, pruritus, irritation, tearing, or eczematous dermatitis.

B. Allergic rhinitis is a reaction of exposure to environmental aeroallergens.

C. Presence of specific-IgE antibody to tested aeroallergens is present in this disease.

II. Epidemiology

A. **About 8–12% of the population is affected with allergic rhinitis**, or about 20–40 million people in the United States.

B. The mean **age of onset is approximately 10 years.**

C. The onset of allergic rhinitis is usually before age 20, and it has a tendency to diminish with time.

D. Allergic rhinitis affects males and females equally.

E. There is a **strong genetic determination.**

F. About 44% of patients with allergic rhinitis may have concomitant nonallergic rhinitis.

III. Pathophysiology

A. Allergic rhinitis is both an **immediate and delayed reaction to airborne allergens,** beginning with the generation and presence of specific antigen-responsive IgE antibody receptors on mast cells of the nasal mucosa.

B. An **antigen-antibody chemical union** begins a series of events in the mast cell, which ends in its degranulation and production of a combination of inflammatory mediators, including histamine, heparin, leukotrienes, prostaglandins, proteases, and platelet-activating factor.

C. An immediate symptomatic response occurs, followed by a more prolonged, **persistent late-phase reaction.** This involves the infiltration into the reactive region of eosinophils, neutrophils, basophils, and mononuclear cells.

IV. Risk Factors

A. Patients with repeated exposure to offending antigens and exposure to multiple offending allergens are at a higher risk of having allergic rhinitis.

B. Patients with other allergies such as atopic dermatitis, asthma, and urticaria are also at a higher risk.

V. Clinical Presentation

A. History of the Patient with Allergic Rhinitis

1. **History of Present Illness**
   a. Nasal stuffiness, congestion, and often paroxysmal sneezing
   b. Watery eyes, sensation of plugged ears, and itchy nose, eyes, ears, and palate
   c. Fatigue and symptom-associated sleeping difficulties
   d. Mouth breathing, scratchy throat, and voice change
   e. Postnasal drip and irritating cough
2. **Past Medical History**
   a. Trauma or facial/sinus surgery (consider cribriform plate fracture)
   b. Polyps
3. **Family History**
   a. Asthma
   b. Rhinitis
   c. Atopic dermatitis
4. **Social and Environmental History**
   a. Occupational exposures
   b. Home exposures
   c. Active and passive smoking exposures
   d. School exposures

B. Physical Examination of the Patient with Allergic Rhinitis

1. **Nose**
   a. **Swollen nasal turbinates** may be boggy, bluish or pale, hyperemic, or purplish red; **note size and color.**
   b. **Clear, cloudy, or colored rhinorrhea;** color can help differentiate between allergic and infectious rhinitis.
   c. There may be **nasal septal deviation or a structural abnormality.**
   d. Nasal polyps
   e. Nasal crease or "salute"
   f. Sneezing
   g. Mouth breathing
   h. Unilateral obstruction may indicate non-allergic rhinitis.
   i. Foreign body may indicate non-allergic rhinitis.
2. **Eyes**
   a. Conjunctivitis
   b. Allergic "shiners" (dark circles under the eyes from venous stasis)
   c. Dennie's lines (lower eyelid creases)
   d. Periorbital edema
3. **Ears:** Acute otitis media or otitis media with effusion suggest associated dysfunction of the eustachian tubes.
4. **Lungs:** Wheezing or prolonged expiratory phase suggest associated asthma.
5. **Skin:** Atopic dermatitis is an associated risk factor for allergic rhinitis.

C. Signs and Symptoms Suggestive of Nonallergic Rhinitis

1. Sensitivity to smoke, perfume, weather changes, and environmental irritants
2. History of previous negative allergy testing

3. Overuse of topical decongestants
4. Adult onset of symptoms
5. Nasal crusting or drying
6. Facial pain

CLINICAL SKILLS TIP

Allergic shiners and clear nasal discharge are commonly associated with allergic rhinitis. Purulent or thickened yellow-green discharge suggests an infectious rhinitis.

VI. Differential Diagnosis (Figure 3–1)

A. Common Diagnoses

1. **Sinusitis:** viral, bacterial, or chronic
2. **Rhinitis:** viral, drug-induced, hormonal, vasomotor, or atrophic or rhinitis medicamentosa
3. Gastroesophageal reflux disease (GERD)
4. Rebound effect associated with continued use of topical decongestant drops and sprays

B. Less Common Diagnoses

1. Systemic disorders such as thyroid disease or Wegener's granulomatosis
2. Nonallergic rhinitis with eosinophilia syndrome (NARES)
3. IgA deficiency with recurrent sinusitis
4. Cribriform-plate defect with cerebrospinal fluid (CSF) leakage (rule out by testing watery discharge for glucose)
5. Chronic aspirin use
6. Overuse of angiotensin-converting enzyme (ACE) inhibitors
7. Septal or anatomic obstruction

RULE OUT

Although allergic rhinitis is the most common cause of clear nasal discharge, a defect in the cribriform plate with CSF leakage must be ruled out if there is suspicion of head trauma. GERD is a common cause of these symptoms, which would not respond to allergic rhinitis therapy but would respond to appropriate therapy if the diagnosis is suspected and confirmed. Consider the diagnosis of GERD if there are other symptoms such as heartburn exacerbated by meals, bending, or recumbency.

VII. Diagnostic Findings

A. **Diagnostic criteria:** The Center for Disease Control (CDC) recommends the following guidelines to avoid the over-diagnosis of sinusitis.

1. Symptoms of rhinorrhea or persistent daytime cough lasting more than 10–14 days without improvement
2. Severe symptoms of acute sinus infection
   a. Fever (> 39° C; 102.2 °F) with purulent nasal discharge
   b. Facial pain or tenderness
   c. Periorbital swelling

B. Laboratory Studies

1. **Complete blood cell count (CBC) with differential:** May show slight increase in eosinophils but often normal if uncomplicated rhinitis.

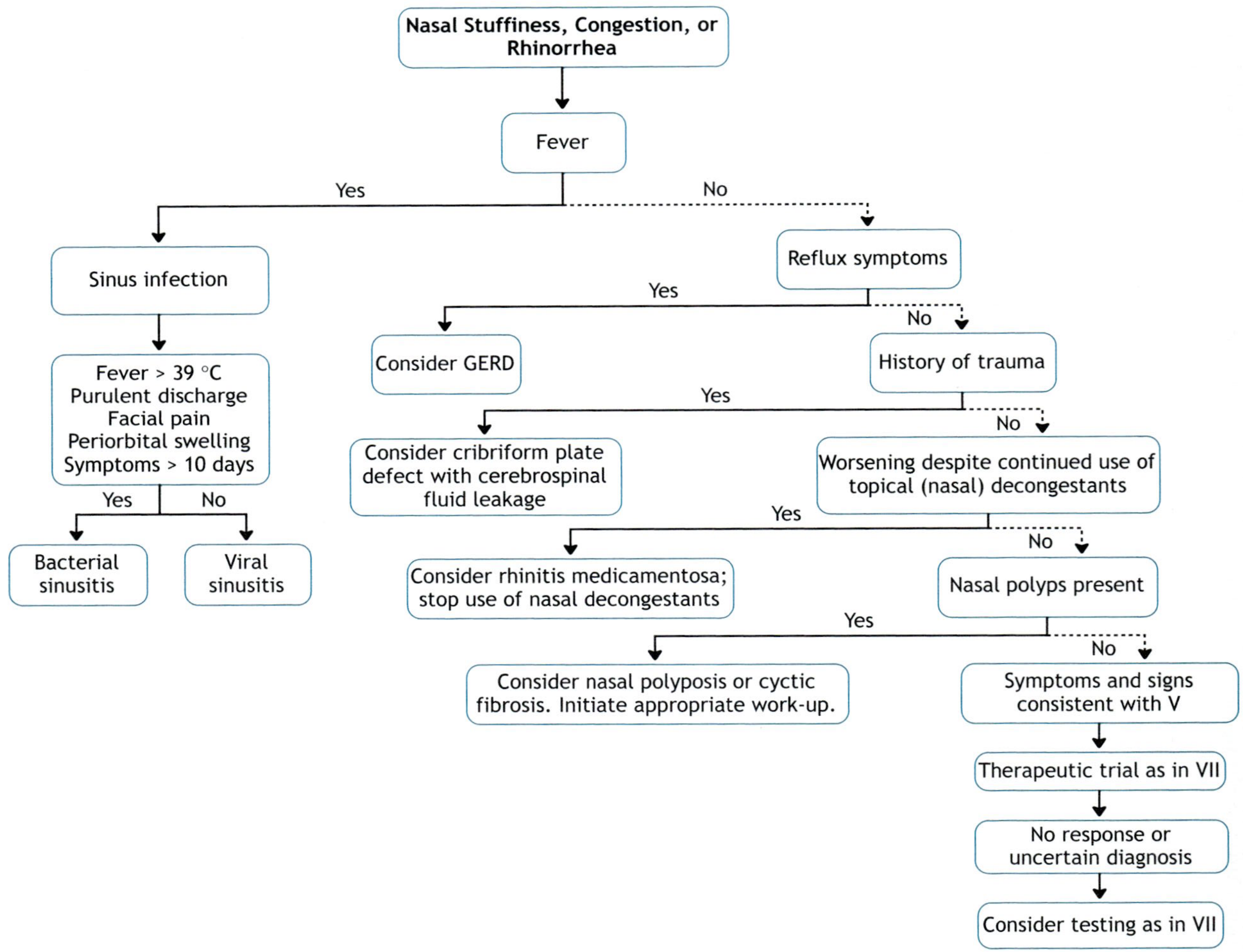

Figure 3–1 Work-up of the patient with nasal stuffiness, congestion, or rhinorrhea.

2. **Nasal Probe Smear with Cytologic Examination for Eosinophils**
   a. **Nasal washing and scraping** will show predominately eosinophils; basophils and mast cells may be seen.
   b. Examination of nasal mucosa will show submucosal edema intact without evidence of destruction. There is eosinophilic infiltration, granulocytes to a lesser extent, an increase in the amount of tissue water with poor staining of ground substance, and congested mucous gland and goblet cells.
3. **Increased IgE level:** Perform radioallergosorbent test (RAST) to determine specific suspected allergens.

C. Diagnostic Procedures

1. **Skin tests** using suspected antigens can be used.
   a. A **scratch or prick skin test** will show a superficial injury to the epidermis with application of diluted test antigen.
   b. An **intradermal skin test** is an introduction of diluted material between layers of skin using a 25- or 27-gauge needle. A 4-mm wheal will demonstrate the patient's response to a susceptible antigen.
2. **RAST** is used, especially in cases where skin testing is not practical (eg, atopic dermatitis and dermatographia).
3. **Audiometry** can be used for deficits and base line evaluation.
4. **Rhinoscopy** is optional but can have excellent visual advantages.

VIII. Treatment

A. **Three classes of pharmacotherapy** are useful in the treatment of IgE-mediated diseases, based on

1. Inhibition of release of mediators from mast cells: **Antihistamines** competitively inhibit the binding of histamine to H_1-receptors and are useful in the treatment of IgE-mediated allergy. Many of these drugs are available over the counter.
2. Inhibition of action of mediators on their target cells: **Sympathomimetic drugs** are useful for their α-adrenergic agonist properties. They can be used orally (eg, pseudoephedrine); topically as nasal decongestants (eg, phenylephrine, naphazoline, oxymetazoline); or topically as conjunctival vasoconstrictors. **Daily use can cause rapid development of rebound vasodilation (rhinitis medicamentosa).**
3. Reversal of the vascular and inflammatory responses in the target tissues: **Glucocorticoids** have a therapeutic role in virtually all types of allergic diseases because of their anti-inflammatory action. They have been proven to greatly reduce nasal symptoms in allergic rhinitis when compared with topical antihistamines. Although available in oral, intramuscular, intravenous, intranasal, and topical formulations for dermatologic use and bronchial inhalation forms, they are currently used mainly in the intranasal form for allergic rhinitis.
4. **Other drugs** acting through various other mechanisms include
   a. **Cromolyn sodium and sodium nedocromil**
   b. **Anticholinergic agents**
   c. **Leukotriene antagonists** have proved to be as effective as antihistamines in improving symptoms of allergic rhinitis.

B. Immunotherapy can also be used in the treatment of allergic rhinitis.

1. Immunotherapy generally should be reserved for **patients with significant allergic rhinitis for whom avoidance measures and pharmacotherapy are insufficient to control symptoms.** The repeated long-term injection of the allergen has been shown to be an effective method to reduce or eliminate symptoms and signs of allergic disorders.
2. Other candidates for immunotherapy include patients who have experienced side effects from medication; those who cannot comply with a regular (or prescribed) pharmacotherapy regimen; or those who develop complications such as recurrent sinusitis.

C. Prevention

1. **Avoidance of the allergen** is the most efficient treatment for any allergic condition. This alleviates the clinical manifestations, but the sensitivity to the allergen will not be reduced.
2. **Pollen** releases occur in the early morning, and the airborne level depends on the wind velocity and temperature. When pollen counts are high, it is helpful to **close windows and stay in air-conditioned environments.**
3. If there is only a slight allergy, keeping the animal out of the bedroom may be sufficient to eliminate **animal danders;** it is usually necessary to remove the animal from the house.
4. To prevent **dust mites,** the mattress and pillows should be **encased in dust mite–proof material.** All bedding should be washed weekly and dried at high temperatures. To prevent **house dust,** rooms should be **dusted frequently** and carpet in the bedroom should be **vacuumed** to help reduce dust. The effectiveness of electronic air purifiers has not proven to help reduce dust mite reduction, because the primary source of exposure is the bed. In sensitized patients, dust mite reduction interventions can be successful adjunctive measures to medical therapy, significantly reduce symptoms, and reduce bronchial hyperreactivity and medication requirements.
5. **Mold spores** are unavoidable outdoors, but activities such as gardening and farming should be avoided because they are associated with acutely high levels of exposure. Indoor mold contamination can be controlled by **repairing leaks, preventing mold buildup** in bathrooms and around windows, and by **replacing mold-contaminated carpeting.**

IX. Summary Table

Condition	Pathophysiology	Diagnostic Studies	Treatment
Allergic rhinitis	Immediate and delayed reaction to airborne allergens	Eosinophils on nasal swab	Antihistamines; sympathomimetic drugs; glucocorticoids; cromolyn sodium and sodium nedocromil; leukotriene antagonists
Sinusitis	Bacterial infection	CBC, imaging and/or polyps on nasal swab	Antibacterials

(continued)

IX. Summary Table (continued)

Condition	Pathophysiology	Diagnostic Studies	Treatment
Viral rhinitis	Viral infection	None	Antihistamines or nothing
Chronic sinusitis	Obstructive process at sinus meatus	None	Antihistamines
GERD	Reflux at esophageal-gastric junction	Consider non-invasive test for *H pylori* infection	Antireflux drugs (see abdominal pain)
Nasal polyposis	Anatomic obstruction	Nasal endoscopy	Antihistamines, possible surgical removal
Hormonal rhinitis	Hormone mediated	None	Antihistamines or none
Rebound effect associated with continued use of topical deconges-tant drops and sprays	Overuse syndrome	None	Discontinue medication
Cribriform plate defect with CSF leakage	Anatomic defect	CT scan of head; test discharge for glucose	Surgical repair

CBC, complete blood cell count; CSF, cerebrospinal fluid; CT, computed tomography; GERD, gastrointestinal reflux disease.

CLINICAL CASE

A 13- year-old girl has had a continuously runny nose for the past 3 months. The discharge has been copious, thin, clear, and watery. Antihistamines have provided only temporary relief. The additional make-up that she has needed to cover the "shiners" under her eyes has been a source of controversy with her family. A recent trial of antibiotics for sinusitis provided only temporary relief as well. She does, however, continue to complain of pressure over her sinuses, which after a school day feels like a headache. At a recent sleepover, her friends accused her of snoring, and this upset her very much. Her past medical history is positive only for recurrent upper respiratory tract infections and ear infections. On physical examination, the girl appears tired. Her eyes are puffy, and her nasal mucosa is boggy. There is some clear, watery discharge from her nose. The remainder of HEENT and physical examinations are noncontributory.

Although allergic rhinitis is a common problem in children, this patient probably presented because of the snoring and because of the conflicts she was having with her parents over the use of make-up. The history is classic for patients with allergic rhinitis. The characteristics of the nasal discharge as well as the shiners and mouth breathing from congestion, which have resulted in snoring, are all common findings. A past history of recurrent upper respiratory tract infections and ear infections is frequently found in patients who have allergic rhinitis. These patients will often be treated empirically for infective sinusitis, although the history is not necessarily consistent. **It is important to differentiate between acute sinusitis and allergic rhinitis to avoid unnecessary prescribing of antibiotics.**

Allergic rhinitis is an antigen-mediated inflammation of the nasal mucosa and may extend into the paranasal sinuses. Diagnosis is usually determined by history and examination ("itchy, running, sneezy, stuffy nose"). A symptom diary and a trial of medication may be helpful to confirm the diagnosis. Allergy testing is rarely helpful and often not needed to confirm the diagnosis, but it may prove to be helpful for patients who have multiple potential allergen sensitivities.

Although the history and physical examination are central to the diagnosis, the physician may choose to conduct diagnostic testing if the results would likely change the management of the patient. As noted above, these tests include skin tests and RAST and nasal smear for eosinophils. CBC for eosinophil count and total serum IgE level generally are not recommended.

Treatment should consist of symptomatic treatment and pharmacotherapy (see VII).

CLINICAL PEARLS

CLINICAL PEARLS

Common findings include nasal stuffiness and congestion; pale, boggy mucous membranes, watery eyes, dark circles under eyes ("allergic shiners,") and mouth breathing.

CHAPTER 4

ASTHMA

I. Defining Features

A. The episodic or chronic symptoms of **airflow obstruction** are breathlessness, cough, wheezing, and chest tightness.

B. The symptoms of airflow obstruction are **usually worse at night** or in the **early morning.** The pattern of symptoms may be either **paroxysmal or constant.**

C. During a physical examination, **prolonged expiratory phase** and **diffuse wheezes** can be heard.

D. During a **pulmonary function test** or **positive bronchoprovocation challenge,** there is limitation of airflow.

E. There is a complete or partial reversibility or airflow obstruction either spontaneously or following **bronchodilator therapy.**

F. **Pulmonary function tests are often abnormal, but the patient has no symptoms.**

II. Epidemiology

A. **Asthma affects approximately 5% of the population, and men and women are equally affected.**

B. About 10 million new cases of asthma are diagnosed each year; however, there is uncertainty about the actual number of cases because of the lack of a uniform definition of the disease.

C. **About 7–19% of cases of asthma are children,** and 50% of the cases are children younger than age 10. It is the leading cause of missed school days (about 7.5 million days per year).

D. There are approximately 470,000 hospital admissions and 5000 deaths per year in the United States.

E. Hospitalization rates are highest among African Americans and children.

F. **Death rates due to asthma are highest among African Americans aged 15–24 years.**

G. Prevalence, hospitalizations due to asthma, and fatalities resulting from asthma have all increased in the United States over the past 20 years.

III. Pathophysiology

A. Asthma is a **disorder of the tracheobronchial tree** and is characterized by mild to severe obstruction to airflow.

B. The histopathologic features include **inflammatory cell infiltration** with neutrophils, eosinophils, and lymphocytes (especially T lymphocytes), mast cell activation, denudation of airway epithelium, collagen deposition beneath the basement membrane, and edema of the airways.

C. All patients will demonstrate **enhanced bronchoconstriction with inhalation of methacholine or histamine.**

D. **Bronchoprovocation studies may show a positive response to inhalation of specific allergens.**

IV. Risk Factors

A. There is a **genetic predisposition** to asthma.

B. **Atopy is the strongest identifiable predisposing factor** for the development of asthma.

C. Asthma symptoms increase with exposure to **environmental tobacco smoke** and cause reduced lung function and the need for increased medications.

D. An increase in airway inflammation, airway hyperresponsiveness, and an increase in symptoms occur with exposure of sensitive patients to inhaled allergens.
   1. **Common aeroallergens** include house dust mites (often found in pillows, mattresses, upholstered furniture, carpets, and drapes), cockroaches, cats, and seasonal pollens.
   2. A **substantial reduction of exposure** reduces pathologic findings and clinical symptoms.

E. Exercise, upper respiratory tract infection, rhinitis, sinusitis, postnasal drip, aspiration, gastroesophageal reflux disease (GERD), atmospheric changes, and stress are some of the nonspecific precipitants of asthma.

V. Clinical Presentation

A. **Symptoms**
   1. Wheezing
   2. Coughing
   3. Dyspnea
   4. Fever
   5. Exercise-induced wheezing or coughing
   6. Nocturnal attacks

B. **Signs**
   1. Prolonged expiration
   2. Tachycardia
   3. Increased use of accessory respiratory muscles
   4. Flattened diaphragms
   5. Growth usually normal

CLINICAL SKILLS TIPS

- *Although a wheeze is a classic and common finding in patients with asthma, a patient may have abnormal pulmonary function tests indicative of asthma even when symptoms are not present. Wheezing may be absent in a patient who has severe asthma in the presence of an acute exacerbation; however, as the patient improves, the wheeze will become more pronounced.*
- *Nocturnal attacks are common due to the delayed phase of the inflammatory response.*
- *As the severity of an acute attack of asthma increases, the use of accessory muscles increases, moving from the sternocleidomastoids to the supraclavicular to the intercostal muscles.*

VI. Differential Diagnosis (Figure 4–1)

A. **Upper airway disorders that mimic asthma** include vocal cord paralysis, vocal cord dysfunction syndrome, foreign body aspiration, laryngotracheal masses, tracheal narrowing, tracheomalacia, and airway edema that occurs in the setting of angioedema or inhalation injury.

B. **Lower airway disorders** include nonasthmatic chronic obstructive pulmonary disease (chronic bronchitis or emphysema), bronchiectasis, allergic bronchopulmonary mycosis, cystic fibrosis, eosinophilic pneumonia, and bronchiolitis obliterans.

C. **Systemic vasculitides** that often have an asthmatic component include Churg-Strauss syndrome and other systemic vasculitides with pulmonary involvement.

D. **Psychiatric causes** of obstructive airways symptoms include conversion disorders (which have been variably referred to as functional asthma), emotional laryngeal wheezing, vocal cord dysfunction, or episodic laryngeal dyskinesis.

E. **Münchhausen syndrome or malingering** may rarely explain the patient's complaints.

RULE OUT

In the presence of a wheeze or airway obstruction, it is important to rule out the presence of an aspirated foreign body or, in an adult, to rule out heart failure.

VII. Diagnostic Findings

A. **Laboratory Studies**

1. Complete blood cell count (CBC) is normal.
2. Smear of nasal secretions shows increased eosinophils.
3. Elevated IgE immunoglobulins are seen in patients who have allergic bronchopulmonary aspergillosis (ABPA).
4. **Perform sweat test in chronic childhood asthmatics to rule out cystic fibrosis (CF).** In absence of CF, sweat test would be normal.
5. **Arterial blood gases** may show hypoxemia and hypercarbia in status asthmaticus.

B. **Imaging studies:** Chest x-ray shows hyperinflation, atelectasis, and air leak.

C. **Diagnostic Procedures**

1. **Spirometry** (pulmonary function testing) includes FEV_1, FVC, and FEV_1/FVC. This test should be performed before and after the administration of a

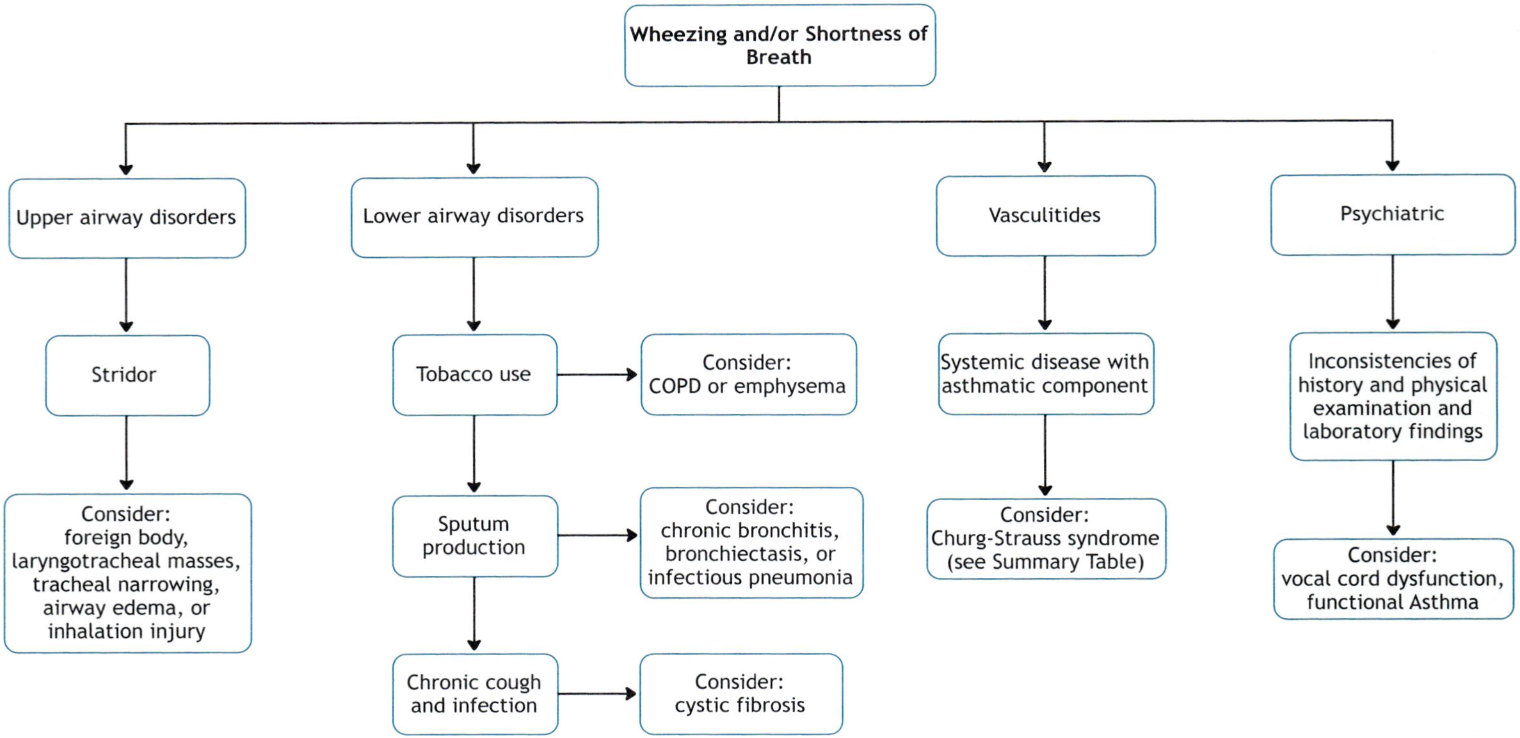

Figure 4–1 Differential diagnosis of obstructive airway disorders other than asthma.

short-acting bronchodilator. **Airflow obstruction is indicated by a reduced FEV_1/FVC ratio (< 75%).**

2. **Bronchoscopy** should be performed if there is a foreign body or a diagnostic uncertainty.
3. **Laryngoscopy** should be performed with exercise challenge to diagnose vocal cord dysfunction.

VIII. Treatment (Table 4–1)

A. Agents Used for Long-Term Control

1. **Anti-inflammatory Agents**
   - a. **Inhaled corticosteroids** are most effective in adults and reduced exacerbations by 55% when compared with placebo. (The National Asthma Education and Prevention Project (NAEPP) statement on inhaled corticosteroids and growth is: Inhaled corticosteroids improve health outcomes for children with mild or moderate persistent asthma, and the potential but small risk of delayed growth is well balanced by their effectiveness.)
   - b. **Systemic Corticosteroids**
2. **Long-acting Bronchodilators**
   - a. Mediator inhibitors
   - b. β-Adrenergic agents
   - c. Phosphodiesterase inhibitors
3. **Leukotriene modifiers** reduced exacerbations by 41% when compared with placebo in adults.
4. **Desensitization**
   - a. **Immunotherapy** may be used in patients who do not respond to environmental control measures. A reduction in acute exacerbations is shown in patients who are treated with single-allergen immunotherapy.
   - b. There is a risk of **immunotherapy-induced bronchoconstriction,** and therefore **immunotherapy should be administered only in a setting where such complications can be treated.**
5. **Miscellaneous Agents**
   - a. Patients who experience bothersome nocturnal symptoms can use oral **sustained-release β_2-agonists.** These agents can also be used for patients who have moderate to severe persistent asthma and who have not responded to other therapies.
   - b. **Corticosteroid-sparing anti-inflammatory agents** include troleandomycin, methotrexate, cyclosporin, intravenous immunoglobulin, and gold and should be used only in selected severe asthmatics.

B. Quick Relief Medications

1. β-Adrenergic agents
2. Anticholinergics
3. Phosphodiesterase inhibitors

C. Prevention

1. The patient should be given an **action plan** and taught to **recognize symptoms.** The action plan should state how the patient should adjust medications in response to particular signs, symptoms, and peak flow measurements and should state when to seek medical help.

Table 4–1. Classification of asthma severity by clinical features before treatment.

Step	Symptoms	FEV_1 or PEF
1. Intermittent	Symptoms less than once a week Brief exacerbations Nocturnal symptoms not more than 2 times a month	FEV_1 or PEF $\geq$ 80% predicted PEF or FEV_1 variability < 20%
2. Mild persistent	Symptoms more than once a week but less than once a day Exacerbations may affect activity and sleep Nocturnal symptoms more than 2 times a month	FEV_1 or PEF $\geq$ 80% predicted PEF or FEV_1 variability 20–30%
3. Moderate persistent	Symptoms daily Exacerbations may affect activity and sleep Nocturnal symptoms more than once a week Daily use of inhaled short-acting β_2-agonist	FEV_1 or PEF 60–80% predicted PEF or FEV_1 variability > 30%
4. Severe persistent	Symptoms daily Frequent exacerbations Frequent nocturnal asthma symptoms Limitation of physical activities	FEV_1 or PEF $\leq$ 60% predicted PEF or FEV_1 variability > 30%

2. **Spirometry** is recommended at the time of initial assessment after treatment is initiated and symptoms and peak flows have stabilized. Spirometry should also be done at least every 1–2 years thereafter.
3. **Regular follow-up visits** (every 6 months) are essential to help maintain asthma control and to re-evaluate medication requirements.
4. The **pneumococcal vaccine** (Pneumovax) and **annual influenza vaccine** should be given to patients who have asthma.

IX. Summary Table

Condition	Pathophysiology	Diagnostic Studies	Treatment
Asthma	Inflammation of conducting airways Bronchospasm increases resistance in all airways	Spirometry	Bronchodilators and anti-inflammatory drugs
Foreign body aspiration	Stridor from inhaled foreign body	CXR and/or endoscopic visualization	Endoscopic removal of foreign body

(continued)

IX. Summary Table (continued)

Condition	Pathophysiology	Diagnostic Studies	Treatment
COPD	Diffuse disease of conducting and lower airways with alveoli destruction	Spirometry, CXR	Bronchodilators and oxygen
Cystic fibrosis	Diffuse disease of conducting airways Physiologic dead space increased	Sweat chloride	Bronchodilators, antibiotics, airway clearance (chest physical therapy, DNAse, flutter device, mucolytic) pancreatic enzymes, nutrition
Vocal cord dysfunction	Emotional stressors and supratentorial etiology	None or laryngoscopy	Emotional/ supportive
Pneumonia	Infection of acini and interstitium	CBC, sputum gram stain CXR	Antibiotics
Systemic vasculitides with pulmonary involvement (eg, Churg-Strauss syndrome)	Vascular inflammatory condition	Need 4 of 6 criteria: Asthma > 10% blood eosinophilia Nonfixed pulmonary infiltrates seen on CXR Paranasal sinus abnormalities Extravascular eosinophils Mononeuropathy or polyneuropathy	Anti-inflammatory drugs and multiple other treatments

CBC, complete blood cell count; COPD, chronic obstructive pulmonary disease; CXR, chest x-ray.

CLINICAL CASE

A 10-year-old boy is brought to the family physician by his mother because she is concerned about the boy's nightly cough. The boy is unaware of the cough, but his mother says that she hears him cough about 5 nights a week. This has been an ongoing pattern for the past 2 months, since school started. The mother says that the cough sounds dry; it is not paroxysmal, and it does not seem that there are periods where the boy is not breathing. Each episode lasts about 1 minute. The boy had a cold 3 months ago, and it has not improved. He has been given antihistamines and decongestants, which have provided minimal to no relief. He is very active at school and plays sports many afternoons. He experiences occasional coughing during or after a game, but it is not significant to him. He is a good student and does well in school. His past history is unremarkable. There is no significant family history other than allergic skin rashes in both parents' families. His physical examination reveals a well nourished and well developed 10-year-old boy. There are no abnormalities in his HEENT, chest, or cardiac examinations.

Although patients can present with status asthmaticus with acute shortness of breath, this presentation of a child with a nocturnal cough is commonly seen in the primary care setting. **The following questions can be helpful when considering the diagnosis of asthma:**

1. Do you have a troublesome cough, particularly at night?
2. Are you awakened by coughing or difficult breathing?
3. Do you cough or wheeze after physical activity?
4. Do you have breathing problems during a particular season?
5. Do you cough, wheeze, or develop chest tightness after exposure to allergens?
6. Do colds "go to your chest" or last more than 10 days?
7. Do you use any medications for your cough? How often?
8. Are your symptoms relieved after you take medication?

Other helpful components include the family history of rashes (ectopy) and the absence of findings consistent with other acute (pneumonia) or chronic diseases (cystic fibrosis). Although school phobias need to be considered for nearly any symptom in a school-aged child, as a good student whose symptoms have not led to school absences, it would be less likely in this case.

This child's nocturnal cough represents the delayed inflammatory response commonly seen in asthma. He plays sports after school and within 6 hours, he coughs as a result of bronchoconstriction and obstruction. Some patients will also describe exercise-induced coughing or wheezing; however, its absence does not rule out asthma as the diagnosis.

Although this patient's physical examination was essentially normal, you could ask the child to run around outside for a few minutes and listen to his lungs after the exercise. You would likely hear a wheeze and prolonged expiration. You could also repeat this maneuver but give him a short-acting bronchodilator before the exercise. Both of these maneuvers would help in determining a diagnosis.

The 4 essential components of asthma management are

1. Assessment and monitoring
2. Controlling factors contributing to asthma severity
3. Pharmacotherapy
4. Education for partnership in care

The first key activity of assessment and monitoring is to establish a diagnosis. Symptomatic adults and children older than age 5 years who have a history suggestive of asthma can be assessed with spirometry. Asthma is indicated with partially reversible airflow obstruction after inhaling a short-acting bronchodilator (> 12% increase and 200 mL of forced expiratory volume in 1 second (FEV_1)). Infants and children younger than age 5 who are unable to perform spirometry should be treated empirically once alternate diagnoses are ruled out.

The next critical activity of the first step is to **classify the severity of asthma.** The patient can be assigned 1 of the 4 steps based on history and peak flow (PEF) or on results of spirometry tests (see Table 4–1).

The second essential component is to identify and control factors contributing to asthma severity. Environmental tobacco smoke (ETS), house dust mites, cockroaches, and cat and dog allergens can worsen asthma (or trigger asthma exacerbations) in sensitized and exposed persons. Irritant or allergen sensitivity can be determined by the patient's exposure and symptom history and confirmed with skin or blood tests. Allergy testing for perennial indoor allergens is recommended for persons with persistent asthma who are taking daily medications. After sensitivity is determined, avoidance of the trigger is recommended, and allergen abatement might be indicated. Examples of trigger avoidance include using pillow and mattress covers that are impermeable to dust mites, removing furry pets, and taking measures to eliminate cockroaches. No patient who has asthma should smoke or be exposed to environmental tobacco smoke. Physicians should review smoking status at the initial visit and at all subsequent visits. If patients smoke or are regularly exposed to environmental tobacco smoke, they should be encouraged to stop smoking and be referred to a smoking cessation program.

The third essential component is pharmacotherapy. Current evidence indicates that daily medications for long-term control are necessary to prevent exacerbations and chronic symptoms for all patients who have persistent asthma, whether the persistent asthma is mild, moderate, or severe. Inhaled corticosteroids are preferred, because they are the most effective anti-inflammatory medication available for treating the underlying inflammation characteristic of persistent asthma. For patients with mild persistent asthma, other long-term medications (ie, cromolyn, leukotriene modifiers, nedocromil, and theophylline) are available but have not been demonstrated to be as effective as inhaled corticosteroids. Patients with moderate or severe disease usually require additional medication in combination with inhaled corticosteroids for daily long-term control. All patients with asthma require a short-acting bronchodilator for managing acute symptoms or exacerbations when they occur; severe exacerbations require the addition of systemic (oral) corticosteroids to treat the increased inflammation present.

The dosage and type of medications are crucial because treatment is adjusted according to the level of severity of asthma. Once therapy goals are achieved, a gradual reduction in treatment should be carefully undertaken to identify the minimum dose required to maintain control (Tables 4–2 and 4–3).

The final essential component is education for partnership in care. As part of the overall management of patients with asthma, the health-care provider, in consultation with the patient or the parent or guardian of a child with asthma, should develop a written plan as part of educating patients regarding self management, especially for patients with moderate or severe persistent asthma and those with a history of severe exacerbation.

Writing the management plan helps clarify expectations for treatment and provides patients with an easy reference for remembering how to manage their asthma. The action plan should include written instructions for recognizing symptoms and signs of worsening asthma; taking appropriate medicines (type, dose, and frequency); recognizing when to seek medical care; and monitoring response to medications. **Symptom-based plans** may be equally effective as plans based on peak flow monitoring, although some patient preferences and circumstances (eg, inability to recognize or report signs and symptoms of worsening asthma) may warrant a choice of peak flow monitoring. The management plan

Table 4–2. Stepwise approach for managing the treatment of infants and young children (age 5 years and younger) who have acute or chronic asthma.

Classify Severity: Clinical Features Before Treatment or Adequate Control		Medications Required to Maintain Long-Term Control
	Symptoms/Day Symptoms/Night	Daily Medications
STEP 4 **Severe persistent**	Continual Frequent	**Preferred treatment:** High-dose inhaled corticosteroids AND Long-acting inhaled β_2-agonists AND, if needed, Corticosteroid tablets or syrup long term (2 mg/kg/day, generally do not exceed 60 mg/day). (Repeat attempts to reduce systemic corticosteroids and maintain control with high-dose inhaled corticosteroids.)
STEP 3 **Moderate persistent**	Daily > 1 night/week	**Preferred treatment:** Low-dose inhaled corticosteroids and long-acting inhaled β_2-agonists OR Medium-dose inhaled corticosteroids **Alternative treatment:** Low-dose inhaled corticosteroids and either leukotriene receptor antagonist or theophylline If needed (particularly in patients with recurring severe exacerbations): **Preferred treatment:** Medium-dose inhaled corticosteroids and long-acting inhaled β_2-agonists **Alternative treatment:** Medium-dose inhaled corticosteroids and either a leukotriene receptor antagonist or theophylline
STEP 2 **Mild persistent**	≥ 2/week but < 1/day > 2 nights/month	**Preferred treatment:** Low-dose inhaled corticosteroid (with nebulizer or MDI with holding chamber with or without face mask or DPI) **Alternative treatment (listed alphabetically):** Cromolyn (nebulizer is preferred or MDI with holding chamber) OR leukotriene receptor antagonist

(continued)

Table 4–2. Stepwise approach for managing the treatment of infants and young children (age 5 years and younger) who have acute or chronic asthma. (continued)

Classify Severity: Clinical Features Before Treatment or Adequate Control		Medications Required to Maintain Long-Term Control
	Symptoms/Day Symptoms/Night	Daily Medications
STEP 1 Mild intermittent	≤ 2 days/week ≤ 2 nights/month	No daily medication needed
Step down: Review treatment every 1–6 months; a gradual stepwise reduction in treatment may be possible.		**Step up:** If control is not maintained, consider step up. First, review patient medication technique, adherence, and environmental control.

DPI, dry powder inhaler; MDI, metered dose inhaler.

Table 4–3. Stepwise approach for managing the treatment of asthma in adults and children older than age 5 years.

Classify Severity: Clinical Features Before Treatment or Adequate Control			Medications Required to Maintain Long-Term Control
	Symptoms/Day Symptoms/Night	PEF or FEV_1 PEF Variability	Daily Medications
STEP 4 Severe persistent	Continual Frequent	≤ 60% > 30%	**Preferred treatment:** High-dose inhaled corticosteroids AND Long-acting inhaled β_2-agonists AND, if needed: Corticosteroid tablets or syrup long term (2 mg/kg/day, generally do not exceed 60 mg/day). Repeat attempts to reduce systemic corticosteroids and maintain control with high-dose inhaled corticosteroids.

(continued)

Table 4–3. Stepwise approach for managing the treatment of asthma in adults and children older than age 5 years. (continued)

Classify Severity: Clinical Features Before Treatment or Adequate Control			Medications Required to Maintain Long-Term Control
	Symptoms/Day Symptoms/Night	PEF or FEV_1 PEF Variability	Daily Medications
STEP 3 **Moderate persistent**	Daily > 1 night/week	≥ 60 % to ≤ 80% > 30%	**Preferred treatment:** Low-to-medium dose inhaled corticosteroids and long-acting inhaled β_2-agonists **Alternative treatment (listed alphabetically):** Increase inhaled corticosteroids within medium-dose range OR Low-to-medium dose inhaled corticosteroids and either leukotriene modifier or theophylline If needed (particularly in patients with recurring severe exacerbations): **Preferred treatment:** Increase inhaled corticosteroids within medium-dose range and add long-acting inhaled β_2-agonists **Alternative treatment:** Increase inhaled corticosteroids within medium-dose range and add either a leukotriene modifier or theophylline
STEP 2 **Mild persistent**	> 2/week but < 1 x/day > 2 nights/month	≥ 80% 20–30%	**Preferred treatment:** Low-dose inhaled corticosteroids **Alternative treatment (listed alphabetically):** Cromolyn, leukotriene modifier, nedocromil, OR sustained-release theophylline to serum concentration of 5–15 mcg/mL

(continued)

Table 4–3. Stepwise approach for managing the treatment of asthma in adults and children older than age 5 years. (continued)

Classify Severity: Clinical Features Before Treatment or Adequate Control			Medications Required to Maintain Long-Term Control
	Symptoms/Day Symptoms/Night	PEF or FEV_1 PEF Variability	Daily Medications
STEP 1 Mild intermittent	$\leq$ 2 days/week $\leq$ 2 nights/month	$\geq$ 80% < 20%	No daily medication needed Severe exacerbations may occur, separated by long periods of normal lung function and no symptoms. A course of systemic corticosteroids is recommended.
Step down: Review treatment every 1–6 months; a gradual stepwise reduction in treatment may be possible.			**Step up:** If control is not maintained, consider step up. First, review patient medication technique, adherence, and environmental control.

should be reviewed and adjusted, as needed, at every visit. For children, a copy of the plan should be given to each care giver and to the child's school.

CLINICAL PEARLS

Wheezing, prolonged expiratory phase, exercise-induced cough or wheezing, and periodicity of symptoms are important findings in diagnosing asthma.

CHAPTER 5
BACK PAIN

I. Defining Features

A. **Back pain is usually a self-limiting condition** of the aging spine.

B. **Lower back pain can result from mechanical stresses and functional demands** placed on the lower back by daily activities.

II. Epidemiology

A. **Back pain is experienced by up to 80% of the United States population.**

B. The lifetime prevalence of patients who experience low back pain is 60–90%. The annual incidence is 5%.

C. About 1% of patients who have acute back pain have symptoms originating in nerve roots.

D. **About 95% of diseased disks are localized to L4–L5 and L5–S1.**

E. Less than 2% of patients with low back pain have infections, neoplasms, or inflammatory spondyloarthropathies.

III. Pathophysiology

A. **Local pain** is caused by activation of local, pain-sensitive nerve endings near the affected part of the spine (eg, tears, stretching).

B. **Pain referred to the back** can be of abdominal or pelvic origin and is unaffected by spinal movement.

C. **Pain of spinal origin** is restricted to the back or referred to the lower limbs. Diseases of the upper lumbar spine refer pain to the upper lumbar region, groin, or anterior thighs. Diseases of the lower lumbar spine refer pain to buttocks or posterior thighs.

D. **Radicular pain** radiates from the spine to the leg in the specific nerve root.

E. **Pain associated with muscle spasm** can have a diverse origin accompanied by taut paraspinal muscles.

IV. Risk Factors

A. Normal aging process (older than age 20)

B. Cigarette smoking

C. Narrow lumbar vertebral canal (for prolapsed disk)

D. Stress and muscle tension
E. Obesity
F. Sedentary lifestyle
G. Vibration (eg, driving motor vehicles)

V. Clinical Presentation

A. Symptoms of Low Back Pain

1. **Onset of low back pain occurs either suddenly after an injury or gradually over the following 24 hours.**
2. Variable pain at the posterior belt line is typically bilateral.
3. Pain occasionally radiates to the buttocks and/or the posterior thighs, stopping at the knees.
4. The pain pattern is referred rather than radicular.
5. Back pain is worse than leg pain.
6. Pain is aggravated by back movement and by sitting, standing, lifting, bending, and twisting.
7. Pain is relieved by rest (recumbency).
8. Bowel and bladder function are preserved.

B. Signs of Low Back Pain

1. **Motor, sensory, and reflex examinations are normal.**
2. There is **decreased lumbar range of motion (ROM) and tenderness** when palpated. Paraspinous musculature spasms are common.
3. Nerve root stretch tests are commonly negative.
4. Tests, including the straight leg raising (SLR) test, that cause spinal motion may increase low back pain but not leg pain.

CLINICAL SKILLS TIPS

Use a sequenced approach following the "4S" positions (Table 5–1). Signs of nerve root involvement such as dermatomal radiation, positive SLR, and other focal neurologic changes will often be present when there is structural disease. Fever, weight loss, loss of appetite, elevated sedimentation rate, or rheumatoid serologies are often present when inflammatory processes are involved. Constitutional symptoms and signs and symptoms referable to a primary tumor will be present when there is referred pain.

VI. Differential Diagnosis

A. Structural

1. Acute or chronic lumbar back pain
2. Low back strain or sprain
3. Herniated lumbar intervertebral disk
4. Degenerative disk disease
5. Spinal stenosis
6. Spondylolisthesis
7. Fractures

B. Inflammatory

1. Ankylosing spondylitis and related inflammatory spondyloarthropathies
2. Infection, including vertebral osteomyelitis, discitis
3. Rheumatoid arthritis

Table 5–1. Physical examination of patients with low back pain sequenced by "4S" positions.

STAND	**1.** Inspect • Lordosis (excess, normal, or decreased), pelvic tilt, kyphosis (osteoporosis), scoliosis • ROM: forward (recheck for thoracic scoliosis), backward, side-bending **2.** Palpate • Paraspinous muscles (spasm?), spinous processes, and interspaces (localized tenderness) • Iliac crest (bilateral pelvic compression) → SI joint pain?
STEPS (walk)	**1.** Gait: symmetry? Antalgic limp (ie, pain-avoiding) **2.** Heel-walking (L4–5), toe walking (S1)
SIT (on exam table)	**1.** Sitting SLR test: should be similar to supine SLR; if not, consider malingering **2.** Strength of quads (L3–4) and ankle plantar flexors (S1), ankle, and large toe dorsiflexors (L5) **3.** Size of calf: measure circumference 10 cm below tibial tubercle **4.** Sensation (circle calf: L3–L5) (circle instep: L4, L5, S1) **5.** Reflexes: knee-jerk (L4), ankle jerk (S1), no "pure" (L5) reflex
SUPINE	**1.** SLR with knee fully extended (180°): Record the angle of hip flexion at which sciatic pain begins; if SLR causes any sciatic pain, try Lasègue's test (SLR with knee at 160°; relaxed hamstrings, dorsiflex ankle): if pain, only with ankle dorsiflexion, Lasègue's test is positive (ie, likely true sciatica) **2.** Hip ROM detects hip flexion deformity **3.** Measure and compare length of legs (anterior superior iliac spine to tip of medial malleolus)

ROM, range of motion; SLR, straight leg raise.

C. Neoplasia

1. Primary tumors
2. Metastases

D. Referred Pain

1. **Orthopedic:** Osteoarthritis of hip
2. **Musculoskeletal:** Sacroiliac joint disease
3. **Gastrointestinal:** Duodenal ulcer, chronic pancreatitis, irritable bowel syndrome, diverticulitis
4. **Genitourinary:** Pyelonephritis, nephrolithiasis, prostatism
5. **Gynecologic:** Pregnancy, endometriosis, ovarian cystic disease, pelvic inflammatory disease
6. **Cardiovascular:** Abdominal aortic aneurysm, vascular claudication

RULE OUT

In adults, the physician should rule out cauda equina syndrome and abscess or infection. In children, look for slipped capital femoral epiphysis (SCFE).

VII. Diagnostic Findings (Figure 5–1)

A. Laboratory Studies

1. Complete blood cell count (CBC) with differential
2. Erythrocyte sedimentation rate (ESR)
3. Alkaline and acid phosphatase
4. Serum calcium
5. Serum protein electrophoresis

B. Imaging Studies

1. **Plain Radiographs**
   a. Not indicated to initiate conservative management program.
   b. Indicated for persistent symptoms of > 1 week duration, patient is older than age 50, or there is a suggestive history.
2. **Radiographs** to rule out tumor or identify other disease process.
3. **Anteroposterior, lateral, spot lateral of L5–S1 and oblique x-rays** and routine **lumbosacral series.**
4. **Bone scan** (scintigraphy) to help identify distinct lesions, osteomyelitis, or systemic bone disease.
5. **Technetium 99m (Tc 99m) pyrophosphate** indicates active mineralization of bone.

C. Diagnostic Procedures

1. **MRI**
2. **CT scan or myelography** is indicated only when there are persistent symptoms, sciatica, or development of neurologic abnormalities.

VIII. Treatment

A. Pharmacotherapy

1. Analgesia can be provided with nonsteroidal anti-inflammatory drugs (**NSAIDs**); severe pain may require opioids.
2. **Muscle relaxants** (eg, diazepam, cyclobenzaprine, carisoprodol, methocarbamol) can be used, but use **only for 1–2 weeks.**

B. Non-pharmacotherapy

1. Patients should be taught how to **protect the back when performing daily activities:** Do not lift heavy objects; use legs rather than back when lifting; use a chair with arm rests; and rise from bed by first rolling to one side and then using the arms to push to an upright position.
2. The **continuation of activities, as tolerated,** is superior to 2 days of bed rest or back-mobilizing exercises.

C. Surgical or Invasive Therapy

1. Patients with a major or evolving neurologic deficit should have a **surgical consultation.** Surgery for disk disease is needed when there is documentation of herniation by imaging, persistent pain, and a consistent neurologic deficit that has failed to respond to 4–6 weeks of conservative therapy.
2. **Epidural corticosteroids** can be used for short-term relief of sciatica, but these drugs do not improve functional status or reduce the need for surgery.

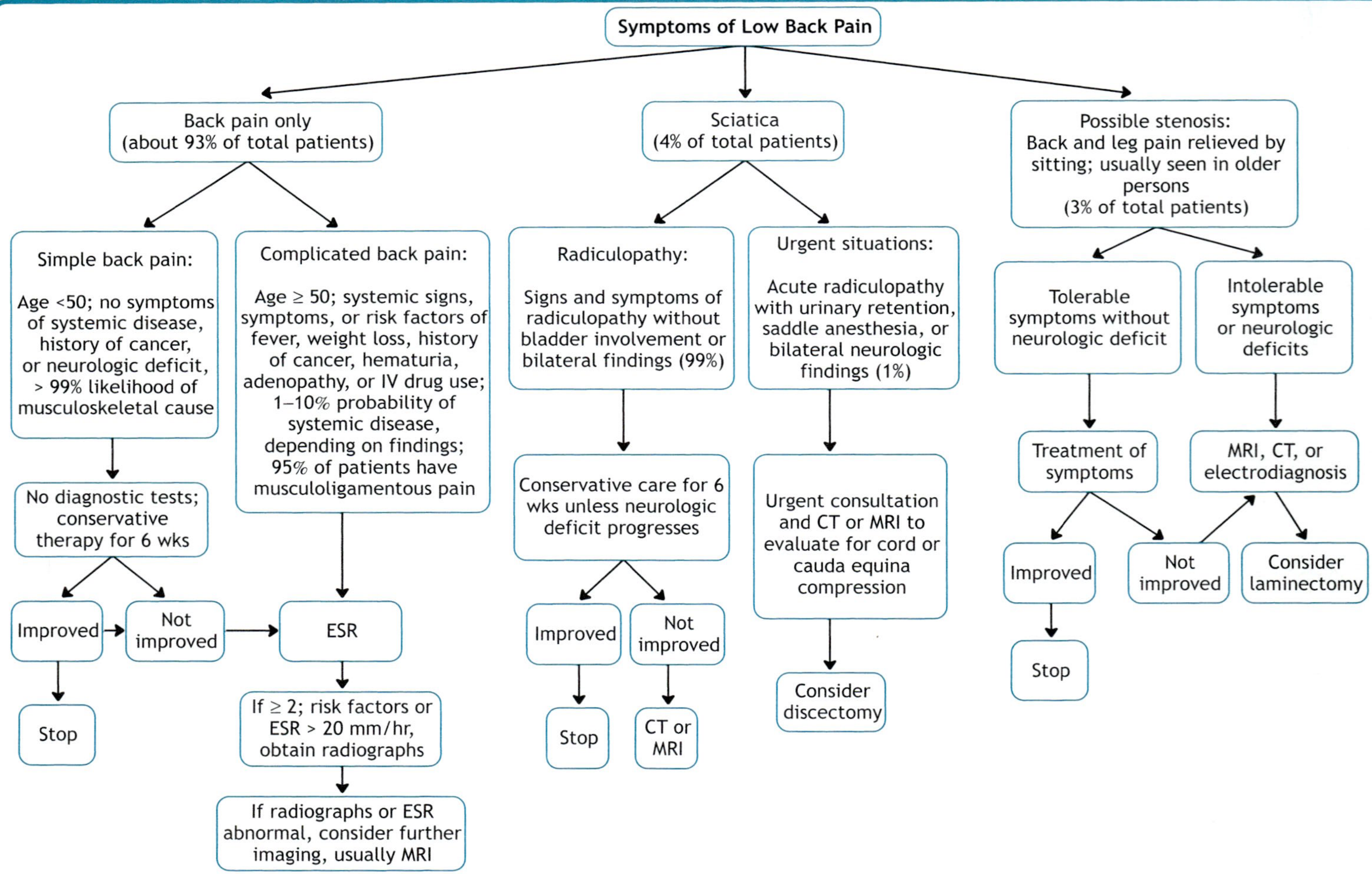

Figure 5–1 Evaluation of the patient with low back pain. Adapted with permission from Jarvik JG, Devo RA. Diagnostic Evaluation of Low Back Pain with Emphasis on Imaging. Ann Internal Med 2002;137: 586–597.

Corticosteroid injections into facet joints are ineffective for chronic low back pain.

3. **Percutaneous lumbar discectomy** is a safe and effective (75%) alternative to laminectomy.

IX. Summary Table

Condition	Pathophysiology	Diagnostic Studies	Treatment
Simple low back pain	Activation of local, pain-sensitive nerve endings	None	Conservative
Spinal infection	Infectious; local or hematogenously spread	CT scan or MRI of spine; CBC; blood cultures	Antibiotics
Spinal tumor	Local or metastatic	CT scan or MRI of spine	As indicated
Sciatica with neurologic involvement	Nerve root impingement	CT scan or MRI of lower spine	Conservative or surgical
Inflammatory/systemic	Rheumatoid arthritis; ankylosing spondylitis; related inflammatory spondyloarthropathies	Lumbar x-rays; CT scan or MRI of spine; serologies; ESR	As indicated by disease

CBC, complete blood cell count; CT, computed tomography; ESR, erythrocyte sedimentation rate; MRI, magnetic resonance imaging.

CLINICAL CASE

A 45-year-old home construction worker has had lower back pain for the past month. He says that about 1 month ago he felt a horrible twisting sensation and heard a pop in his lower back when he was moving a stack of dry wall. This was followed almost immediately by pain. After resting his back for 3 days, he returned to work. He has continued working, although he has low back pain nearly every day. He describes the pain as sharp and rather severe on both sides of his lower back. The pain was originally on his left side, but it now seems to be on both sides. When asked, he rates the pain as a 6 on a scale of 1 to 10. He is able to do his work, but he is tired of being in pain. Although he feels the pain mainly in his lower back, he occasionally feels pain down his left leg to his mid-thigh. He has had no fever. Although he is tired, he does not think that he has weakness in his legs. He denies loss of bowel or bladder function. He takes no medications other than ibuprofen or acetaminophen, which he takes every night before going to bed so he can sleep. Toward the end of the interview, he mentions that he thinks he just cannot continue doing construction work anymore. His past medical history is noncontributory. He drinks about 1 six-pack of beer on Friday and Saturday nights. He does not use tobacco or illegal drugs. He is divorced and lives alone. On physical examination, he appears tired. His vital signs and HEENT, heart, and lung examinations are all normal. Examination of his back reveals decreased lumbar ROM and tenderness to palpation of his paraspinous musculature. There is also spasm of the paraspinous muscles. SLR test increases his lower back pain, but there is no leg pain. The remainder of his neurologic examination is normal, including deep tendon reflexes and motor and sensory testing.

The differential diagnosis for this patient is extensive. Important considerations include cancer, spinal infection, cauda equina, and neurologic involvement when there is sciatica. **Risk factors for cancer** include

1. Age 50 years or older
2. History of cancer (concern for metastasis)
3. Unexplained weight loss
4. Failure to improve after 4–6 weeks of conservative low back pain therapy

If all 4 of these risk factors are absent, cancer can be ruled out with 100% sensitivity.

Risk factors for spinal infection include IV drug use and urinary retention. Patients using IV drugs are also at risk for infectious endocarditis and may have intermittent low-grade fevers. Work-up should proceed with an MRI of the lower spine and CBC and blood cultures.

Signs and symptoms of cauda equina syndrome include urinary retention, saddle anesthesia, unilateral or bilateral sciatica, and sensory and motor deficits. Patients with these symptoms require immediate MRI.

Patients with sciatica will have signs and symptoms of radiculopathy. The pain will radiate down the leg below the knee. Concerning findings in these patients include

1. Urinary retention
2. Saddle anesthesia
3. Bilateral neurologic findings

Patients with these symptoms must have immediate consultation and CT scan or MRI to evaluate for cord or cauda equina compression. Weakness or numbness in the legs with sciatica radiation beyond the knee raises concern for neurologic involvement. If the patient does not improve with conservative treatment, immediate MRI is required.

Patients with spinal stenosis are generally older patients. Classically, their back and leg pain is relieved by sitting. If they have intolerable symptoms or neurologic deficits, an MRI, CT scan, or electrodiagnosis must be performed to confirm the suspicion of spinal stenosis.

It is important to examine the patient's psychosocial history. Is there a history of substance abuse, failed previous attempts at treatment, or requests for disability compensation? These patients are challenging, and guidelines for their management will not be considered here.

Our patient's presentation is extremely common in primary care offices. He has **simple, uncomplicated back pain**. Differentiating simple from complicated back pain in patients with back pain involves only the following criteria used to diagnose complicated back pain:

1. Age older than age 50
2. Systemic signs or symptoms
3. Fever
4. Weight loss
5. History of cancer
6. Hematuria
7. IV drug use

There is a > 0.99% likelihood that simple back pain will have a musculoskeletal cause. Nearly 95% of patients with complicated back pain will have musculoligamentous pain. Acute and chronic low back pain is differentiated by duration: acute pain is < 6 weeks and chronic pain is > 6 weeks.

Although our patient is extremely bothered by his pain, he has no worrisome signs or symptoms and it is still < 6 weeks since the pain began (**6 weeks is a useful cut-off as a guideline for treatment**). This case mentions that the neurologic examination was normal and non-focal. It is important to include the following components in this examination:

1. Ankle dorsiflexion strength
2. Great toe dorsiflexion strength
3. Ankle reflexes
4. Knee reflexes
5. Sensory exam with pinprick sensation in the medial, dorsal, and lateral aspects of the foot
6. SLR test should be assessed bilaterally to evaluate for nerve root impingement, including but not limited to disk herniation. Positive SLR is defined as pain in the posterior leg, which radiates below the knee with the patient lying supine and the hip flexed ≤ 60°, is suggestive of disk herniation. Negative SLR rules out surgically significant disk herniation in 95% of cases.

Other than the urgent consultations mentioned above, patients with simple, uncomplicated low back pain do not require any laboratory or imaging investigations. Most patients will improve within 2 weeks, and most will experience significant improvement within 4 weeks. **Conservative home care** should include

1. Early ambulation.
2. Limited bed rest.
3. Gentle stretching and modified sit-ups as part of a daily regimen.
4. Apply ice and heat to the sore area to lessen inflammation (short duration).
5. Take anti-inflammatory and analgesic over-the-counter medications.
6. Early return to work.

The above home care regimen should be recommended to our patient whose symptoms have been present < 6 weeks. If he returns without improvement, an ESR is recommended. If it is > 20 mm/h, lumbar radiographs should be ordered. If the radiographs are abnormal, evaluation should proceed to imaging, usually MRI.

With conservative treatment, follow-up is important. Ask the patient to return for a follow-up visit within 1–3 weeks. It is important for the patient to know that more than half of the patients who recover from a first episode of acute low back symptoms will have another episode within a few years. Unless the back symptoms are very different from the first episode or the patient has a new medical condition, expect improvement quickly from each episode.

CLINICAL PEARLS

Most patients have benign disease without neurologic impairment. In the absence of worrisome findings, 6 weeks of conservative therapy is appropriate. MRI imaging should be done immediately in patients with symptoms of cauda equina syndrome.

CHAPTER 6
CHEST PAIN

I. Defining Features

A. **Precordial chest pain** is usually precipitated by exertion or stress and is relieved rapidly by rest or by nitrates.

B. Evidence of **ischemia** during pain or stress testing can be seen on an electrocardiogram (ECG).

C. Significant obstruction of major coronary vessels can be seen on an angiogram.

II. Epidemiology

A. **Angina** is the presenting symptom of coronary heart disease in 38% of men and 61% of women.

B. **Angina is most common in middle-aged and older men and in postmenopausal women.**

III. Pathophysiology

A. Angina results from an imbalance between myocardial oxygen supply and demand, most commonly resulting from **atherosclerotic coronary artery obstruction.**

B. There may be no abnormal physical examination findings.

IV. Risk Factors

A. Family history of premature coronary artery disease (CAD)

B. Hypercholesterolemia

C. Hypertension

D. Tobacco abuse

E. Diabetes mellitus

F. Male gender

G. Advanced age

H. Morbid obesity

V. Clinical Presentation (Figure 6–1)

A. Symptoms of Angina

1. **Precordial pressure or heaviness** may be brought on by exercise, emotional stress, eating large meals, inhaling cold air, or smoking and is relieved by rest or nitrates.

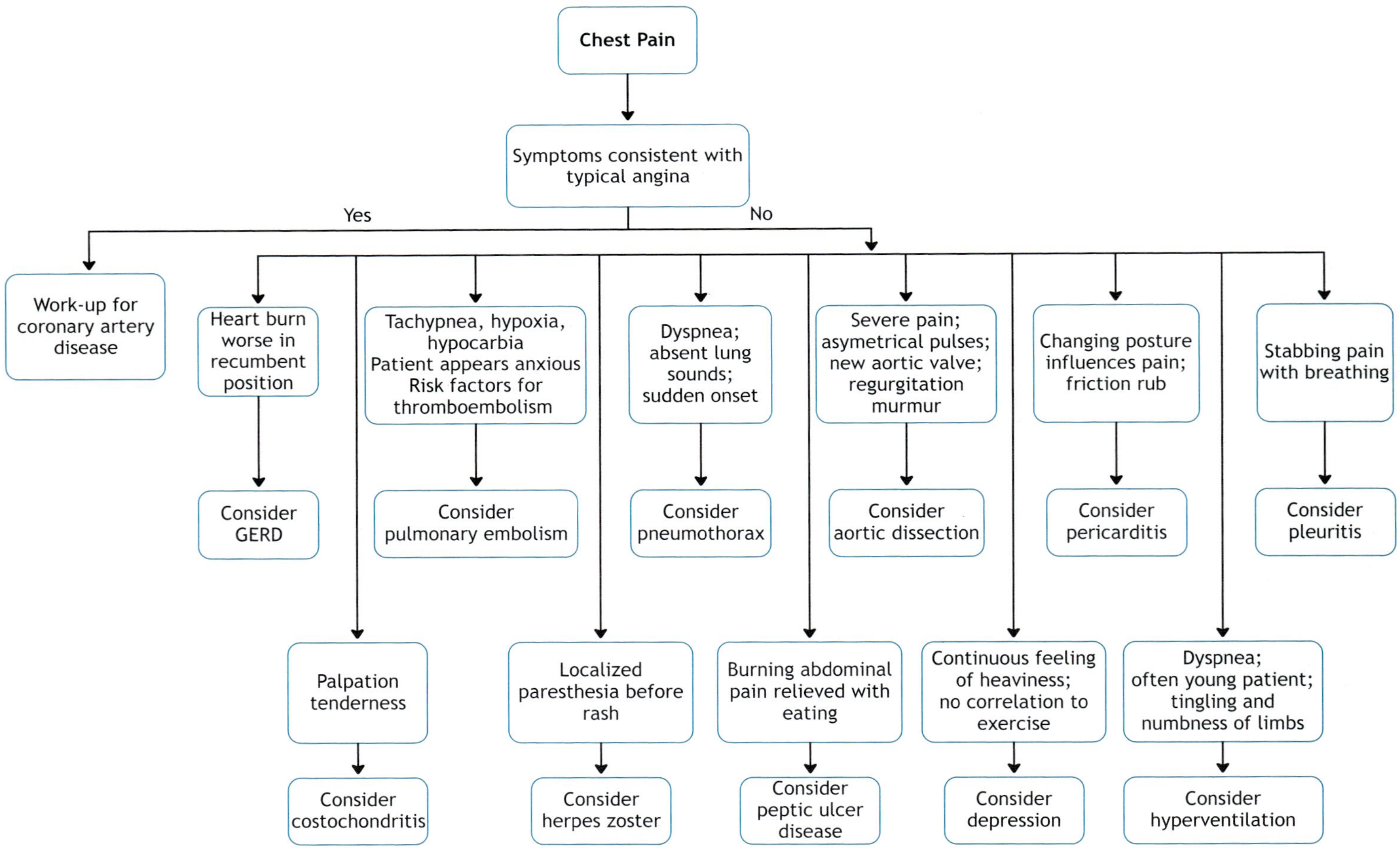

Figure 6–1 Differential diagnosis of chest pain.

2. The pain is described as a **sensation of a tight band around the chest;** breathing or changing posture does not notably influence the severity of the pain.
3. Discomfort may be described by the patient with a clinched fist over the sternum (Levine's sign).
4. The **duration of pain is usually > 20 minutes;** it is continuous and its intensity does not alter.
5. **Dyspnea on exertion may present as the only symptom.**
6. **A choking sensation on exertion is a classic symptom.**
7. **Discomfort or pain may radiate** to the neck, lower jaw, teeth, shoulders, and inner aspects of the arms or back.
8. **Pain beginning in the upper abdomen** with nausea may resemble the symptoms of acute abdomen. **Nausea and vomiting** are sometimes the main symptoms, especially in inferoposterior wall ischemia.

B. **Signs of Angina**

1. **Tachycardia, tachypnea, hypo- or hypertension** may indicate impaired left ventricular function.
2. **S3 or S4 sounds** may indicate ventricular volume overload or impaired compliance.
3. **Pulmonary crackles or râles** may indicate impaired cardiac output from infarction.

CLINICAL SKILLS TIPS

Irritation of the central portion of the diaphragm, either the pleural or peritoneal surfaces, causes pain at the superior border of the trapezius muscle and the supraclavicular fossa. Stimulation of either surface of the peripheral portions of the diaphragm causes pain in dermatome T6. Dermatomes T1–T6 form a band that covers most of the thorax and extends down the anteromedial aspect of the arms and forearms. Sensory pathways from the viscera of this region are so interconnected that stimulation of any area can produce the same patterns of chest pain.

VI. Differential Diagnosis (see Figure 6–1)

A. **Anterior chest wall syndrome** is characterized by sharply localized tenderness of the intercostal muscles. Inflammation of the chondrocostal junctions, which may be warm, swollen, and red, may result in diffuse chest pain that is also reproduced by local pressure.

B. **Cervical or thoracic diseases of the spine** can be confused with angina, because cervical or thoracic also produces chest pain. This pain occurs only with specific movements of the neck and spine, recumbency, and straining and lifting and involves the outer or dorsal aspect of the arm and the thumb and index fingers.

C. **Gastroesophageal reflux disease (GERD)** may result in chest pain that is characterized by lower chest and upper abdominal pain and occurs after eating large meals. This pain occurs in recumbency or when bending over. It can awaken patients several hours after eating.

D. **Degenerative and inflammatory lesions** of the left shoulder and thoracic outlet syndromes may cause chest pain. This pain is due to nerve irritation or muscular compression and is usually associated with movement of the arm and shoulder.

E. **Spontaneous pneumothorax** causes chest pain on the affected side.

F. **Myocardial infarction** (MI) causes chest pain that often radiates to the neck or down the left arm.

G. **Pneumonia** causes sharp or stabbing chest pain that is worsened by deep breathing or coughing.

H. **Pulmonary embolism** can cause sharp or stabbing chest pain. The pain may also be burning, dull, or aching.

I. **Dissection of the thoracic aorta** causes severe chest pain that is sudden, stabbing, and tearing.

J. **Pericarditis** may produce chest pain with postural changes.

RULE OUT

In the presence of angina, it is important to rule out an acute MI, dissecting aortic aneurysm, or pulmonary embolism. These are all life-threatening conditions, and their timely diagnosis is critically important.

VII. Diagnostic Findings

A. **Laboratory Studies**

1. **Total cholesterol** is typically **elevated.**
2. **HDL** cholesterol is typically **reduced.**
3. **LDL** cholesterol level is typically **elevated.**

B. **Imaging Studies**

1. **Radionuclide angiography** images the left ventricle and measures its ejection fraction and wall motion. In coronary artery disease (CAD), resting abnormalities usually represent infarction, and those that occur only with exercise usually indicate stress-induced ischemia. Patients who have CAD may exhibit a decrease in ejection fraction with exercise.
2. **Coronary angiography** can visualize the location and severity of stenoses and can show whether the obstructions are amenable to bypass surgery or to percutaneous transluminal coronary angioplasty.
3. **Myocardial perfusion scintigraphy** can provide information about the presence, location, and extent of coronary artery disease. If the radiotracer is injected during exercise or dipyridamole or adenosine-induced coronary vasodilation, the scintigraphy scan demonstrates a zone of hypoperfusion that may represent either ischemia or scar.
4. **Positron emission tomography (PET)** can demonstrate either perfusion or metabolism of the myocardium.
5. **Echocardiography** images the left ventricle and reveals segmental wall motion abnormalities, which may indicate ischemia or prior infarction. When this test is performed during supine exercise or immediately following upright exercise, it can show exercise-induced segmental wall motion abnormalities as an indicator of ischemia.

C. **Diagnostic Procedures**

1. **CT scan** can image the heart and assist in the evaluation of pericardial disease.
2. **Cardiac MRI** can show left ventricular functions and wall motion.
3. **Ambulatory electrocardiographic monitoring** can detect rhythm abnormalities not shown during a single 12-lead ECG.
4. **Resting ECG** is normal in about 25% of patients with angina.

VIII. Treatment

A. Pharmacotherapy

1. **Sublingual nitroglycerin** acts in about 1–2 minutes. This drug can also be taken 5 minutes before any activity likely to precipitate angina.
2. **Nitrates** decrease arteriolar and venous tone, reduce preload and after load, and reduce the oxygen demand of the heart. They also improve myocardial blood flow by dilating collateral channels and, in presence of increased vasomotor tone, coronary stenoses.
3. **Morphine sulfate** can be used in the acute setting for pain that does not respond to nitroglycerin. Such patients need to be evaluated for the presence of an acute MI.

B. Prevention

1. **Reduce risk factors** by reducing LDL, treating hypertension, stopping smoking, and introducing exercise and a weight loss program.
2. Hypertension, left ventricular failure, arrhythmia, strenuous activity, cold temperatures, and emotional states can all aggravate angina.
3. **β Blockers** can help prevent angina by reducing myocardial oxygen requirement during exertion and stress.
4. **Calcium-channel blocking agents,** including verapamil, diltiazem, and the dihydropyridine group, are agents that can help prevent angina.
5. **Platelet-inhibiting agents** are beneficial following unstable angina and infarction. **A dose of baby aspirin** (81 mg) can be prescribed for patients with angina.
6. **Revascularization** may be indicated for
   a. Patients who have unacceptable symptoms despite medical treatment.
   b. Patients who have left main artery stenosis > 50% with or without symptoms.
   c. Patients who have 3 vessels that are diseased and ejection fraction < 50%.
   d. Patients who have unstable angina who continue to exhibit ischemia on exercise testing.
   e. Post-MI patients who have continuing angina or severe ischemia on noninvasive testing.

IX. Summary Table

Disease	Pathophysiology	Diagnostic Studies	Treatment
Coronary artery disease/angina	Myocardial O_2 demand > supply	ECG, ETT, angiography	NTG, O_2
MI	O_2 deficit to myocardium resulting in muscle death	ECG, angiography	O_2, ASA 160 mg, MSO_4, β blocker

(continued)

Summary Table (continued)

Disease	Pathophysiology	Diagnostic Studies	Treatment
GERD	Acid refluxing into distal esophagitis	EGD	PPI, H_2-blocker
Spontaneous pneumothorax	Air leakage into pleural space	CXR or CT scan of thorax	100% O_2
Pulmonary embolism	Obstruction in pulmonary vasculature leading to O_2 deficit	Spiral CT scan of thorax, D-dimer	Thrombolytics
Cervical or thoracic spine disease	Bone or local irritation of spinal nerves	X-ray of cervical or thoracic spine, CT scan	NSAIDs
Dissecting aortic aneurysm	Intimal tear of artery leading to O_2 loss distally	CT scan of thorax	Surgery
Pneumonia	Infectious process in lung	CXR	Antibiotics

ASA, acetaminophen; CT, computed tomography; CXR, chest x-ray; ECG, electrocardiogram; EGD, esophagogastroduodenoscopy; ETT, exercise tolerance test; GERD, gastroesophageal reflux disease; MI, myocardial infarction; NSAID, nonsteroidal anti-inflammatory drug; NTG, nitroglycerin; PPI, proton pump inhibitor.

CLINICAL CASE

A 48-year-old man comes to see you complaining of chest pain that he has had for the past 2 days. Recently, he has been particularly active playing tennis, and he thought it was a strain from playing. He has not played tennis or any other sport for the past few years. Currently, he is not experiencing any pain. He tells you that the pain first occurred 2 days ago during the first set of a tennis game when he was serving. He thought it was due to the stretching involved with serving and tried to ignore it. When he experiences the pain, it lasts about 15 minutes in the retrosternal area. The pain goes down his left arm. He says that he assumed the pain of a strain would go down his left arm because he is left dominant. When asked, he tells you that the pain felt heavy, almost tight and band-like around his chest. He felt somewhat nauseous, which he attributed to the game and heat. When the game was over, he and his friends sat in the shade and rested and the pain went away. The next day, he and his friends began to play earlier in the day. He took ibuprofen when he got home on the previous day and *again on the morning before he left for the courts. After he began playing, he experienced pain exactly like that he had the previous day. He quit playing, and his friends urged him to go to the hospital but he said that he felt fine and took more ibuprofen. This morning he has no pain, but his family insisted that he see you for an evaluation. He continues to tell you that it was only a strain. His past history is noncontributory since he never sees his physician. He takes no medications. He has had no surgeries. His father died in his early 40s, possibly from heart disease. He smokes tobacco, but has cut down from 2 packs a day to 1½ packs a day. He generally has 1 or 2 beers with his friends after work. He denies using illegal drugs. He is divorced and currently is not sexually active. He does not think that he has ever had his cholesterol tested. He says that he frequently eats fast food since his divorce. On physical examination, his blood pressure is 158/92 mm Hg (with the large cuff), and his pulse is 86 and regular. His BMI is 32.5. His HEENT is noncontributory. There is no jugular venous distention. His pulmonary examination is normal and there are no crackles. His heart has a normal point of maximal impulse (PMI) and normal S_1 and S_2. There are no murmurs. His abdomen is obese. The remainder of his physical examination is normal. An ECG performed on presentation reveals a normal sinus rhythm and no ST or T wave abnormalities.*

This patient has at least 2 concerning diagnoses: CAD and denial. On presentation to the office or emergency department, the physician must differentiate the patient with CAD from the patient with non-coronary chest pain. Non-coronary causes of chest pain that are nonetheless urgent and require rapid triage include pulmonary embolism, spontaneous pneumothorax, aortic dissection, and pericarditis. The list of less urgent non-cardiac causes of chest pain is extensive (Table 6–1). Our patient has a classic description of chest pain associated with CAD (see I A).

Table 6–1 Non-cardiac causes of chest pain.

Condition	Differentiating symptoms & signs
GERD, esophageal spasm	No ECG changes Heartburn Worse in recumbent position, but also while straining Most common cause of chest pain
Hyperventilation	Hyperventilation syndrome includes • Main symptom is dyspnea • Often a young patient • Tingling and numbness of limbs and dizziness • Decreased $PaCO_2$; increased or normal PaO_2 Secondary hyperventilation: • Attributable to organic illness or cause: acidosis, pulmonary embolism, pneumothorax, asthma, infarction
Pleuritis	Stabbing pain when breathing

(continued)

Table 6–1 Non-cardiac causes of chest pain. (continued)

Condition	Differentiating symptoms & signs
Costochondral pain	Pain influenced by palpation, tenderness, movements of the chest May also be an insignificant incidental finding
Early herpes zoster	No ECG changes; rash; localized paresthesias before rash
Ectopic beats	Transient in the area of the apex
Peptic ulcer, cholecystitis, pancreatitis	Clinical examination is critical
Depression	Continuous feeling of heaviness in the chest; no correlation to exercise; normal ECG
Alcohol-related	Often seen with young inebriated person in ED

ECG, electrocardiogram; ED, emergency department; GERD, gastroesophageal reflux disease.

A critical task for the physician is triage. Patients with cardiac ischemia should be triaged to a hospital emergency department. The primary care physician must focus the patient's treatment on prevention as well as on pharmacologic management of the CAD. For those patients who have chronic stable angina or those who are asymptomatic but who have evidence of CAD, **medical management** should include

1. Aspirin
2. β Blocker
3. Angiotensin-converting enzyme (ACE) inhibitor
4. Statin, if cholesterol level is above normal

Prevention activities should focus on modifiable risk factors, including tobacco use, exercise, obesity, and diet. Cigarette smoking is the most important cause of preventable morbidity and early mortality. Exercise can increase HDL and help with weight loss. Although the impact of dietary modifications on total cholesterol serum levels may be limited, it allows patients to exert more control over their disease.

CLINICAL PEARLS

Although the characteristics of cardiac chest pain are classic, the physician must triage among the non-cardiac causes of worrisome chest pain, cardiac chest pain, and the non-worrisome causes of non-cardiac chest pain.

CHAPTER 7
CONTRACEPTION

I. Defining Features

A. Contraception is used to **prevent unwanted pregnancies.**

B. **Methods of Contraception**
1. Oral contraceptive pills (OCP)
2. Contraceptive injections
3. Other hormonal methods: transdermal patch and vaginal ring
4. Intrauterine devices (IUD)
5. Diaphragm and cervical cap
6. Contraceptive foam, cream, film, sponge, jelly, and suppository
7. Condom
8. Contraception based on awareness of fertile periods
9. Emergency contraception (EC)
10. Abortion
11. Sterilization: vasectomy and laparotomy

II. Epidemiology

A. About two thirds of women at risk for unwanted pregnancies use some type of contraception.

B. Contraceptives are used by females from menarche through menopause and by males after they reach puberty.

C. In 1995, 62.4% of women aged 15–44 years used some method of contraceptive.

D. Oral contraceptive pills (OCPs) were the most common form of contraception used in 1995.

III. Pathophysiology

A. The **progestin-estrogen combination** pill effectively inhibits secretion of follicle-stimulating hormone (FSH) and lutein hormone (LH) from the pituitary, thus preventing follicular development in the ovary and ovulation.

B. **Other contraceptive effects of the progestin-estrogen preparations** include alteration of the endocervical mucus and the endometrial mucosa to create a hostile environment for the passage of sperm and nidation of the fertilized embryo.

C. One form of oral contraceptive contains **progestin only,** the so-called **"mini-pill."** This single-agent contraceptive was introduced to avoid the complications associated with the use of estrogen.

IV. Risk Factors

A. Risk factors associated with contraceptive use include cardiovascular complications (OCPs); pelvic inflammatory disease (IUDs); depression and weight gain (progestin-only contraceptives); and vaginal and urinary tract infections (barrier methods).

B. The risk factor for pregnancy is that **any woman who is ovulating and who engages in intercourse with a fertile male is at risk of becoming pregnant.**

C. **Adolescents and those of lower socioeconomic class** with less education about reproduction have a greater risk of becoming pregnant.

CLINICAL SKILLS TIP

The physician is allowed to discuss contraception at any visit with patients of child-bearing age.

V. Contraceptive Options

A. Oral Contraceptive Pills (OCPs)

1. The OCP is taken on the first or fifth day of the ovarian cycle and taken daily for 21 days, followed by 7 days of inactive pills to maintain a 28-day pill cycle.
2. **OCPs have a failure rate of less than 0.5%** if always taken on schedule.
3. There are many different types of pills but, essentially, there is no clinically significant difference.
4. The **benefits of oral contraceptives** include lighter menstrual flow; anemia is less common; dysmenorrhea is relieved; functional ovarian cysts disappear; pain with ovulation and postovulatory aching are relieved; risk of ovarian and endometrial cancer is decreased; risk of salpingitis and ectopic pregnancy can be diminished; acne improves; myomas develop less often; and there is a beneficial effect on bone mass.
5. **OCPs can have a decrease in efficacy when taken concomitantly with phenytoin, phenobarbital, primidone, carbamazepine, or rifampin.**
6. **Adverse effects** of OCPs include myocardial infarction, thromboembolic disease, cerebrovascular disease, carcinoma, metabolic disorders, hypertension, headache, amenorrhea, and disorders of lactation.

B. Contraceptive Injections and Implants

1. The injectable hormone **progestin medroxyprogesterone acetate** is approved for contraceptive use in the United States.
   a. The **hormone is injected every 3 months** and has a 99.7% efficacy rate.
   b. **Common side affects** include irregular bleeding, amenorrhea, weight gain, and headaches.
2. A **monthly injectable hormone containing both depot medroxyprogesterone acetate and an estrogen** is available in the United States.
3. **Norplant** is a longer acting implant contraceptive that is **no longer available in the United States.**

C. Other Hormonal Methods

1. A **transdermal contraceptive patch** containing 150 μg **norelgestromin** and 20 μg **ethinyl estradiol** and measuring 20 cm^2 is available. The patch is applied to the lower abdomen, upper torso, or buttock once a week for 3 consecutive weeks, followed by 1 week without the patch.

2. A **vaginal ring** that releases 120 μg of **etonogestrel** and 15 μg of **ethinyl estradiol** daily is available. The ring is placed in the upper vagina for 3 weeks, removed for 1 week, and then replaced with a new ring.

D. Intrauterine Devices (IUDs)

1. **Mirena** and **copper-bearing TCu380A** IUDs are available in the United States.
2. IUDs contain **spermicidal or inhibitory effects** on sperm capacitation and transport.
3. **Contraindications and complications** associated with IUDs include pregnancy, pelvic infection, acute or subacute pelvic inflammatory disease or purulent cervicitis, menorrhagia or severe dysmenorrhea, and complete or partial expulsion.

E. Diaphragm and Cervical Cap

1. The **diaphragm is a dome-shaped rubber cup** that must be inserted with a spermicide before coitus and must remain in place at least 6 hours after coitus.
    a. The diaphragm has **no systemic side effects** and offers significant protection against pelvic infection and cervical dysplasia as well as against pregnancy.
    b. **Failure rates** of the diaphragm are **2–20%.**
2. The **cervical cap** covers only the cervix and can be more difficult to insert and remove than the diaphragm.

F. Contraceptive Foam, Cream, Film, Sponge, Jelly, and Suppository

1. These products are all **available without prescription,** are easy to use, and are fairly effective, **with failure rates of 2–30%.**
2. All of these products contain the spermicide **nonoxynol-9.**

G. Condom

1. Condoms provide protection against pregnancy, sexually transmitted diseases (STDs), and cervical dysplasia.
2. Disadvantages of male condoms include dulling of sensation and spillage of semen due to tearing, slipping, or leakage, with detumescence of the penis. The **failure rate is 3–12%.**
3. A female condom is also available with **failure rates of 5–21%.**

H. Contraception Based on Awareness of Fertile Periods

1. There are methods in which to identify the times when the woman is most fertile, and unprotected intercourse should be avoided during these times.
2. **Symptothermal natural family planning** is a contraceptive approach when the woman looks for signs that she is fertile, including an increase in clear elastic cervical mucus, brief abdominal midcycle discomfort, and a sustained rise of basal body temperature. To avoid pregnancy, unprotected intercourse should be avoided when these changes are occurring.
3. With the **calendar method,** a woman observes the length of her menstrual cycle and calculates the days on which she is most fertile. Based on normal menstrual cycles (28 days), a woman is most fertile on approximately day 14, with day 1 being the first day of the last menstrual period (or 14 days before the menstrual period).
4. With the **basal body temperature contraceptive method,** a woman takes her temperature daily upon awakening. There is a slight decrease in body

temperature 12–24 hours before ovulation and an increase of about 0.4 °C 1–2 days after ovulation.

I. Emergency Contraception (EC) (Table 7–1)

1. **Levonorgestrel** (prepackaged in the United States as Plan B) can be given in 2 doses 12 hours apart to prevent pregnancy **after unprotected intercourse.**
2. **Ethinyl estradiol,** 50 μg, with 0.5 mg **norgestrel** (prepackaged in the United States as Preven), can be **taken after unprotected intercourse.**
3. **Ethinyl estradiol** is an effective emergency contraception; however, it has a higher likelihood of producing **side effects of nausea, vomiting, and breast tenderness.**

Table 7–1. Emergency contraception available in the United States.

Trade Name	Pills Per Dose & Color of Pill	Ethinyl estradiol Per Dose (μg)	Levonorgestrel Per Dose (mg)
Ovral**¶	2 white pills	100	0.50
Alesse	5 pink pills	100	0.50
Levlite	5 pink pills	100	0.50
Nordette**	4 light-orange pills	120	0.60
Levlen**	4 light-orange pills	120	0.60
Levora	4 white pills	120	0.60
Lo/Ovral*¶	4 white pills	120	0.60
Triphasil**	4 yellow pills	120	0.50
Tri-Levlen**	4 yellow pills	120	0.50
Trivora	4 pink pills	120	0.50
Ovrette¶	20 yellow pills	0	0.75
Dedicated products			
Preven§ ||	2 blue pills	100	0.50
Plan B||	1 white pill	0	0.75

**These products were declared safe and effective for use as emergency contraception by the FDA in February 1997. The other products listed are bioequivalent.

¶—The progestin in Ovral, Lo/Ovral, and Ovrette is norgestrel, which contains two isomers, only one of which (levonorgestrel) is bioactive; the amount of norgestrel in each tablet is twice the amount of levonorgestrel.

§— Preven comes with a pregnancy test kit.

||—Both Plan B and Preven are labeled by the FDA for emergency contraceptive use

J. Abortion

1. Since abortion became legal in the United States in 1973, the related maternal mortality rate has dropped because of the decrease in illegal and self-induced abortions and because abortions are now performed using safer medical procedures.
2. About **90% of abortions are performed before 12 weeks' gestation.**
3. **Complications from legal abortions** include retained products of conception and unrecognized ectopic pregnancy.

K. Sterilization

1. Couples who no longer want children most often choose sterilization as the most acceptable method of birth control.
2. **Vasectomy (male sterilization)** is a procedure in which the vas deferens is severed and sealed through a scrotal incision.
3. **Laparotomy or tubal ligation (female sterilization)** is currently performed via laparoscopic bipolar electrocoagulation, via application of a plastic ring on the uterine tubes, or via minilaparotomy with Pomeroy tubal resection.

RULE OUT

When a woman comes to her physician requesting contraception, the most important rule out is that she currently is not pregnant. Although the currently available urine hCG has a sensitivity of 50 IU, within approximately the first 6 days after intercourse, this test will not yet be positive. It is during this time that the physician cannot reliably ascertain the patient's pregnancy status.

VI. Diagnostic Procedures during Family Planning Visit (Figures 7–1 and 7–2)

A. Females

1. **Cervical cytology:** Pap test
2. **Cultures for gonorrhea and chlamydia**
3. **Blood lipids and blood glucose**
4. **Pregnancy test** (if hormonal contraception is not initiated at time of menses)

B. Males

1. There are no diagnostic procedures except routine preoperative studies prior to vasectomy.
2. Semen analysis after vasectomy; aspermia requires up to 15 ejaculations.

CLINICAL CASE

A 21- year-old woman comes to see you urgently on Monday morning. Although the chief complaint is listed as "check-up," your nurse tells you that the patient said that she had unprotected intercourse the previous night. She has been a regular patient of yours for 10 years. As she begins to tell you her story, it is clear that she is upset. She has had an off-again, on-again relationship with a male friend since she left for college 3 years ago. She is home on vacation and after spending time with her friend, they had unprotected intercourse < 24 hours ago. She confirms that no alcohol or drugs were involved and there was no violence. She tells you that it was consensual sex. She has no complaints at this time or any symptoms. Her parents are aware of her relationship with the fellow, and she has told them about the sexual encounter the previous

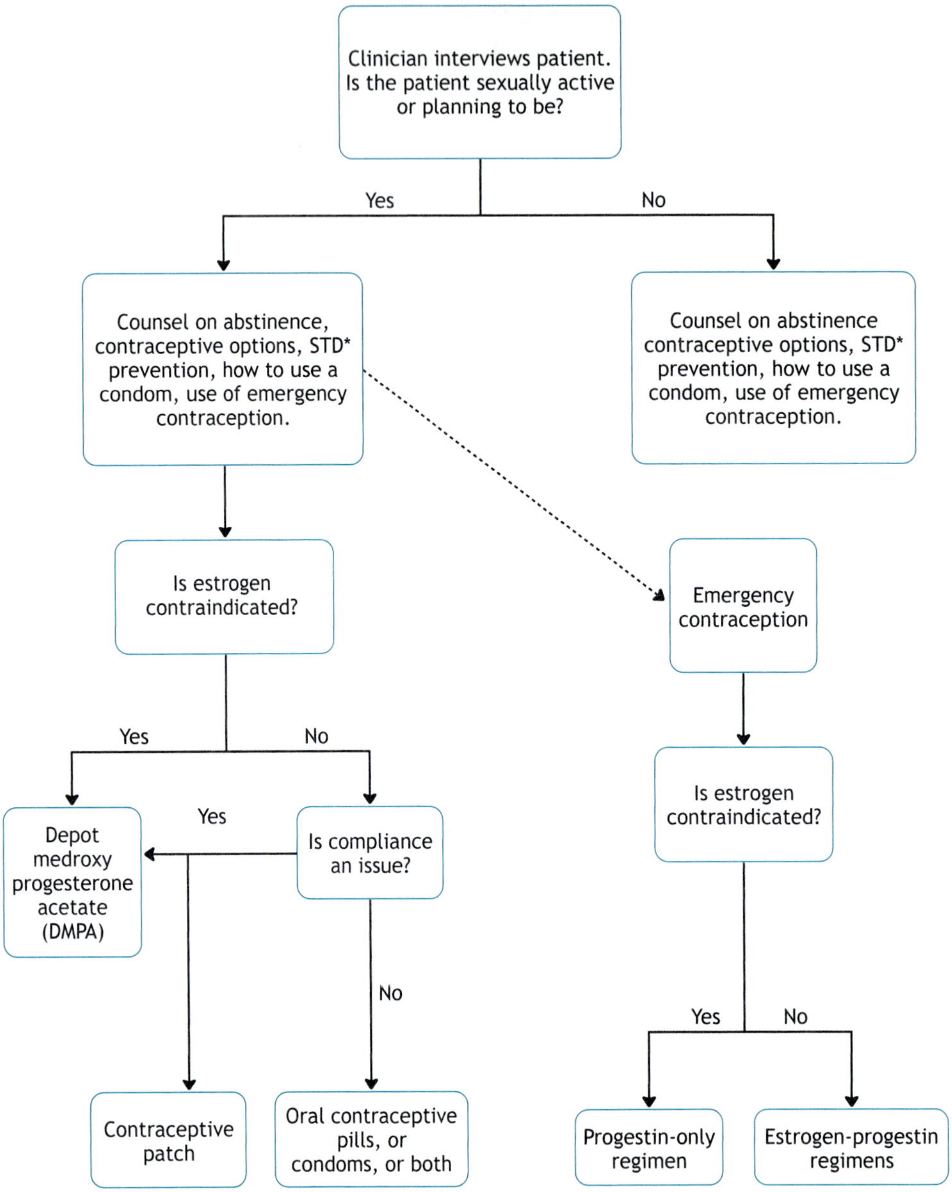

* STD, Sexually transmitted disease

Figure 7–1 Initiating contraception.

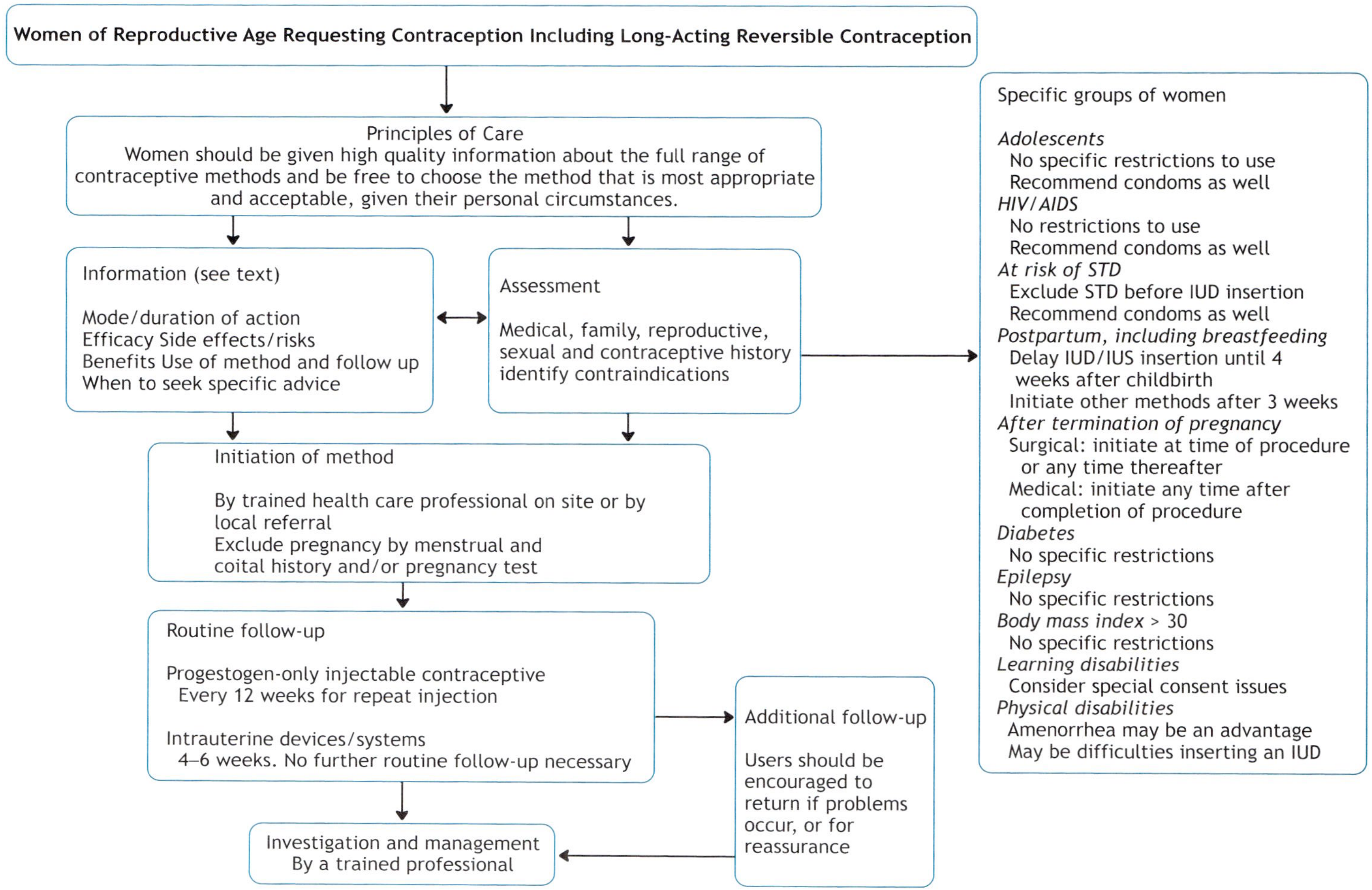

Figure 7–2 Effective and appropriate use of long-acting reversible contraception.

evening. She has had intercourse 2 times previously with the same man, and on both occasions he used a condom. She had intended to go to the campus health service to request information about contraceptive options, but her relationship with the fellow ended and she decided not to go. Her past history is otherwise unremarkable. During her last visit with you nearly 4 years ago, you administered a complete history and provided a meningococcal vaccine. She has never had a pelvic examination or a Pap smear. She asks for a prescription for emergency contraception. She readily acknowledges that it is time for her to discuss ongoing contraceptive options. Her vital signs are within normal limits. You do not perform a physical examination at this time.

This is a relatively common presentation to physicians who care for young adults. In communities where there are Planned Parenthood offices, many young women use these services. Sometimes patients are worried about confidentiality and will avoid their family physician because they fear that their parents will be told about the visit. Our patient has an open relationship with her parents and has already informed them about the sexual encounter. If a patient comes to see you and has not discussed this topic with her parents, your role is to maintain a confidential relationship with your patient. However, you should encourage your patient to speak openly with her parents, and you could offer to facilitate that discussion.

Emergency contraception has long been an option, and there are now drugs that are specifically labeled by the FDA for use as an emergency form of contraception. Previously, various doses of OCPs could be used as emergency contraception. OCPs can still be used; however, there are 2 products specifically labeled for this use (see V I and Table 7–1). Guidelines regarding emergency contraception published by the American College of Obstetrics and Gynecology (ACOG) in 2001 include

1. **Combination or progestin-only** oral contraceptives for emergency contraception should be offered to women **within 72 hours of having unprotected sexual intercourse.**
2. Because the **progestin-only** method produces less nausea and may be more effective than the combination oral-contraceptive method, this regimen **should be strongly considered.**
3. To minimize nausea and vomiting with combination oral-contraceptive products, an **antiemetic agent should be prescribed** and the patient should take it 1 hour before the first dose of oral contraceptive.
4. During a routine gynecologic visit, physicians who wish to increase the availability and use of emergency contraception may offer patients an advance prescription for emergency contraception.

Although a scientific panel recommended that Plan B status be changed to over-the-counter availability, the FDA rejected this recommendation in 2004. Therefore, this patient must see you (the physician) to receive the Plan B drug.

To use EC pills, 2 doses must be taken 12 hours apart. The first dose should be taken as soon as possible after intercourse, and the second dose should be taken 12 hours after the first dose. The most common side effects are nausea and, to a lesser extent, vomiting. Plan B and other progestin-only pills are reported to cause less nausea and vomiting than the combined formulas. Taking an over-the-counter anti-nausea medication 1 hour before the first EC dose can greatly reduce these side effects. If a woman does vomit within 2 hours of taking her first dose, she should contact a health care provider. It is important to take only the amount of pills prescribed. Taking more pills than prescribed will not decrease a woman's chance of getting pregnant, but it will increase the chance of experiencing nausea and vomiting. Other less common side effects are breast tenderness, headaches, menstrual irregularities, and dizziness.

EC pills work in various ways. They may inhibit or delay ovulation, alter the tubal transport of sperm or the egg (thereby preventing fertilization), or alter the lining of the uterus, which may inhibit the implantation of a fertilized egg. If a woman is already pregnant when she takes EC pills, they will not harm the fetus. Emergency contraception is contraception, not abortion. It prevents pregnancy before it occurs.

After discussing the options with our patient, she chooses Plan B. You ask her to make a follow-up visit to your office to discuss ongoing contraception. At the follow-up visit, it is important to recognize that although there are many contraceptive options whose efficacy is outstanding, the effectiveness of each option is determined by the patient. You must work with her to find the option that she is willing to use consistently and correctly. This decision will often be based on the patient's personal beliefs, preferences, and specific needs at the time. Your role is to educate the patient about the advantages and disadvantages of each method that is medically appropriate for her, and then allow her to choose the most desirable method that she wishes to use. It is critically important to differentiate between birth control and protection against STDs. This visit provides an excellent opportunity to perform a Pap test.

Although the list of available contraceptive options is long, it is reasonably easy to narrow the list after an initial discussion with your patient. In the past few years, this list of options has expanded and a few options are no longer available. The combined hormonal vaginal ring releases 15 mcg of ethinyl estradiol and 120 mcg of etonogestrel daily. It remains in the vagina for 3 weeks and then is removed. After 1 ring-free week, a new ring is inserted by the patient. The contraceptive patch works similarly to OCPs but requires only 1 weekly application by the patient. It releases 20 mcg of ethinyl estradiol and 150 mcg of norelgestromin a day. After 3 weekly patches, there is a patch-free week during which withdrawal bleeding occurs. There is also a new intrauterine system that releases levonorgestrel. It provides similar efficacy to the traditional intrauterine devices but is associated with less menorrhagia and dysmenorrhea. There is a combined hormonal injection that requires monthly injections rather than every 3 months as occurs with the progestin-only injection. Although it is FDA-approved, it currently is not manufactured for use in the United States. A combination OCP that contains the new progestogen drospirenone has been available for the past few years. Drospirenone has some antimineralocorticoid activity and has been shown to decrease the water retention and appetite changes that are associated with changes in the menstrual cycle. The FDA has approved the use of levonorgestrel-ethinyl estradiol combination in an extended OCP regimen consisting of 84 days of active pills and 7 days of nonhormonal pills (Tables 7–2 and 7–3).

CLINICAL PEARLS

When unprotected intercourse occurs, patients may consult their physicians regarding options. This visit provides an opportunity to discuss contraception.

Table 7–2. Contraceptive options.

Method	Mechanism of Action	Patient Selection Criteria	Absolute Contraindication to Use	Side Effects	Non-contraceptive Benefits	Potential Complications
OCPs	Inhibits ovulation by suppressing FSH & LH Increases transit time of egg through fallopian tubes Thickens cervical mucous	Effectiveness depends on patient compliance	Undiagnosed vaginal bleeding History of breast cancer or other estrogen-dependent cancer Active liver disease History of MI, stroke, DVT, PE, heavy smoking in women > 35 years or smoking in women > 40 years	Increased risk of cardiovascular disease in smokers and with increased age HTN Nausea, headaches, dizziness, spotting, weight gain, breast tenderness Amenorrhea or irregular bleeding	Decreases menstrual pain, premenstrual syndrome, and blood loss; protects against symptomatic PID, against some cancers (ovarian, endometrial), against some benign tumors (leiomyomata, benign breast masses), and against ovarian cysts; reduces acne	Cardiovascular complications (stroke, heart attack, blood clots, hypertension); depression; hepatic adenomas; possible increased risk of breast and cervical cancers
IUD	Creates a local inflammatory response that lyses the blastocysts/sperm Prevents implantation by increasing local prostaglandins	Women in a mutually monogamous relationship and low risk for acquiring STDs No history of ectopic pregnancy Not indicated in nulliparous women	History of repeated STDs Women with history of ectopic pregnancy	Menstrual cramping, spotting, increased bleeding Expulsion Perforation of uterine wall	Copper-containing IUDs may provide protection against endometrial cancer; progesterone-releasing IUDs decrease menstrual blood loss and pain	PID (following insertion), uterine perforation, anemia
Male condom				Decreased sensation, allergy to latex, loss of spontaneity	Protects against STDs, including HIV infection; delays premature ejaculation	Anaphylactic reaction to latex

Female condom				Aesthetically unappealing; may be awkward to use	Protects against STDs	None known
Hormonal implant	Inhibits ovulation Thickens cervical mucus to inhibit sperm penetration	Women who want to delay childbearing for several years but want rapid return of fertility Effective, long-term method Women with a contraindication to estrogen Adolescents	Active thrombophlebitis Undiagnosed vaginal bleeding Active liver disease Known or suspected breast cancer Benign or malignant liver tumor Decreased efficiency in women taking rifampin, phenobarbital, or other antiseizure drugs	Tenderness at implant site, menstrual irregularities, hair loss, weight gain	Does not disturb lactation; may decrease menstrual cramps, pain, and blood loss	Infection at implant site, complicated removal, depression
Progestin-only injections	Inhibits ovulation resulting in increased FSH & LH Thickens cervical mucus Makes endometrium unsuitable for implantation	Women who have difficulty remembering to take meds Women who have completed childbearing but do not want sterilization Women who have contraindication to estrogen or OCPs	Active thrombotic problems Active liver disease Undiagnosed vaginal bleeding History of stroke, MI or breast cancer	Unpredictable menses, weight gain, headaches, adverse effects on cholesterol levels (ie, decreases HDL level) Weight gain Decreased libido	Does not disturb lactation; reduces risk of seizures; may have protective effects against PID as well as ovarian and endometrial cancers	Depression, allergic reactions, pathologic weight gain; possible bone loss

(*continued*)

Table 7–2. Contraceptive options. (continued)

Method	Mechanism of Action	Patient Selection Criteria	Absolute Contraindication to Use	Side Effects	Non-contraceptive Benefits	Potential Complications
Female sterilization	Surgical procedure where fallopian tubes are ligated or cauterized	Women who have completed childbearing	None	Pain at surgical site; psychologic reactions, including regret that procedure was performed	Reduces risk of ovarian cancer; may protect against PID	Infection, anesthetic complications; if pregnancy occurs after tubal ligation, high risk of ectopic pregnancy
Abstinence	No intercourse leading to meeting of sperm and egg	Patient choice	Patient reliability	Psychologic reactions	Prevents STDs, including HIV infection	None known
Barrier contraceptives: diaphragm, cervical cap, vaginal sponge	Kills sperm or blocks their entry into the cervical os	Effectiveness depends on patient compliance	None	Pelvic pressure, vaginal irritation, allergy; vaginal discharge if left in too long Increased incidence of UTIs	Provides modest protection against some STDs	Vaginal and urinary tract infections; toxic shock syndrome

Spermicides	Kills sperm or blocks their entry into the cervical os	Effectiveness depends on patient compliance	None	Vaginal irritation, allergy to foam or jelly	Provides modest protection against some STDs; potential increased risk of HIV infection with use of nonoxynol-9	Vaginal and urinary tract infections
Lactational amenorrhea	Presumed inhibition of ovulation through lactation	Early postpartum, however reliability is limited	None	Mastitis from staphylococcal infection	Breast-feeding has nutritional benefits for infant	Increased risk of HIV transmission to infant if mother is HIV positive

DVT, deep vein thrombosis; FSH, follicle-stimulating hormone; HDL, high density lipoprotein; HTN, hypertension; HIV, human immunodeficiency virus; IUD, intrauterine device; LH, leuteinizing hormone; MI, myocardial infarction; OCP, oral contraceptive pill; PE, pulmonary embolus; PID, pelvic inflammatory disease; STD, sexually transmitted disease; UTI, urinary tract infection.

Table 7–3. Overview of contraceptive options currently available in the United States.

Contraceptive Method	Unintended Pregnancies Within First Year of Use (%)		Women Continuing Use at 1 year (%)	Protection Against STDs
	Typical use*	Perfect use†		
None	85	85	—	—
Spermicide	29	15	42	No§
Withdrawal	27	4	43	No
Periodic abstinence				
Calendar method	25	9	~ 50	No
Ovulation method	25	3	~ 50	No
Symptothermal method ‖	25	2	~ 50	No
Post-ovulation method	25	1	~ 50	No
Cervical cap: parous women¶	32	26	46	No
Cervical cap: nulliparous women¶	16	9	57	No
Diaphragm¶	16	6	57	Yes#
Female condom	21	5	49	Yes
Male condom	15	2	53	Yes
OCPs	8	0.3	68	No
Contraceptive patch	Unknown	0.3	68	No
Vaginal ring	Unknown	0.3	68	No
Progestin-only OCPs	3	0.3	56	No
Copper-containing IUD	0.8	0.6	78	No
Levonorgestrel intrauterine system	0.1	0.1	81	No

(*continued*)

Table 7–3. Overview of contraceptive options currently available in the United States. (continued)

Contraceptive Method	Unintended Pregnancies Within First Year of Use (%)		Women Continuing Use at 1 year (%)	Protection Against STDs
	Typical use*	Perfect use†		
Female sterilization	0.5	0.5	100	No
Male sterilization	0.15	0.10	100	No

STD = sexually transmitted disease; OCP = oral contraceptive pill; IUD = intrauterine device;
*—Among typical couples who initiate use of a method (not necessarily for the first time), the percentage who experience an accidental pregnancy during the first year if they do not stop use for any other reason.
†—Among couples who initiate use of a method (not necessarily for the first time) and who use it perfectly (both consistently and correctly), the percentage who experience accidental pregnancy during the first year if they do not stop use for any other reason.
§—Possible decrease in human papillomavirus transmission but no protection against HIV infection, gonorrhea, and chlamydial infection; potential increase in HIV transmission with use of nonoxynol-9.[11]
||—Cervical mucus (ovulation) method supplemented by calendar method in preovulatory phase and by basal body temperature method in postovulatory phase.
¶—Method used with spermicide.
#—May protect against gonorrhea, chlamydial infection, cervical dysplasia, and pelvic inflammatory disease; protection against HIV infection cannot be assumed.
Adapted from Hatcher RA. A pocket guide to managing contraception. 5th ed. Tiger, Ga.: Bridging the Gap Foundation, 2000-2003:36, 44–141.

CHAPTER 8
COUGH

I. Defining Features

A. Patients seek care due to **prolonged cough.**

B. **Dyspnea associated with the cough** will often lead patients to seek care.

C. **Tobacco use and other environmental pollutants** often lead to cough.

II. Epidemiology

A. The most common causes of cough are bronchitis, the common cold, and laryngotracheobronchitis (LTB).
   1. **Bronchitis** occurs among **all age groups.**
   2. **Cough due to the common cold is more predominant in children** than adults.
   3. **LTB affects mostly children and boys** more often than girls. Its prevalence is 15,000–40,000/100,000.

B. A **chronic cough** can affect all age groups, and there is a prevalence of 14–23% in nonsmokers.

C. American Indians and Inuits are at a higher risk of getting common colds and having subsequent complications than are other ethnic groups.

III. Pathophysiology

A. Cough is a result of **stimulation of mechanical or chemical afferent nerve receptors** in the bronchial tree.

B. **Inflammatory cough** occurs as a result of **edema and hyperemia** of airways and alveoli due to laryngitis, tracheitis, bronchitis, bronchiolitis, pneumonitis, or lung abscess.

C. **Mechanical cough** is caused by **inhalation of particulates** (dust) or **compression of airways** (eg, pulmonary neoplasms, foreign bodies, granulomas, bronchospasm).

D. **Chemical cough** is caused by **inhalation of irritant fumes** (eg, cigarette smoke).

E. **Thermal cough** is caused by **inhalation of cold or very hot air.**

IV. Risk Factors

A. Infants and older persons

B. Smoking tobacco, second-hand smoke, and air pollutants

C. Exposure to infected persons

D. Environmental changes and bronchopulmonary allergies
E. Gastroesophageal reflux disease (GERD)
F. Chronic bronchopulmonary diseases and chronic sinusitis
G. Alcoholism
H. Recurrent upper respiratory tract infections (URIs) and history of croup
I. Hypertrophied tonsils and adenoids in children
J. Immunoglobulin deficiency
K. Immunosuppression
L. Stress

V. Clinical Presentation

A. Signs and Symptoms of Bronchitis

1. **Preceding respiratory tract infection** (eg, common cold with coryza, malaise, chills, slight fever, sore throat, back and muscle pain)
2. **Cough,** initially dry and unproductive, then productive subsequently with mucopurulent sputum
3. Fever
4. Fatigue and aching
5. Hemoptysis
6. Burning feeling in chest
7. Rales, rhonchi, wheezing
8. Absence of pulmonary consolidation
9. Pharynx injected (appears red)

B. Signs and Symptoms of the Common Cold

1. Nasal stuffiness and/or obstruction
2. Sneezing
3. Scratchy throat
4. Cough
5. Hoarseness
6. Malaise
7. Headache
8. Temperature > 100 °F (37.7 °C)

C. Signs and Symptoms of Laryngotracheobronchitis

1. Barking, spasmodic cough
2. Biphasic stridor
3. Low-grade to moderate fever
4. URI prodrome lasting 1–7 days
5. Hypoxia/cyanosis
6. Fatigue
7. Non-toxic appearing child
8. Normal voice, no drooling

CLINICAL SKILLS TIP

The clinical examination, including use of office spirometry or peak flow testing, can be extremely helpful in the evaluation of the patient with cough. Consider peak flow testing with provocation (have the patient run around the block) and after use of bronchodilator therapy.

VI. Differential Diagnosis (Figures 8–1 and 8–2)

A. Bronchitis

1. Asthma or reactive airways disease
2. Influenza
3. Bronchopneumonia
4. Acute sinusitis
5. Aspiration or retained foreign body
6. Bacterial tracheitis
7. Inhalation injury
8. Heart failure
9. Bronchogenic carcinoma

B. Common Cold

1. Mumps
2. Rubeola
3. Allergic rhinitis
4. Cytomegalovirus
5. Epstein-Barr virus
6. *Mycoplasma pneumoniae*
7. Influenza

C. Laryngotracheobronchitis

1. Epiglottitis
2. Foreign body aspiration
3. Subglottic stenosis (congenital or acquired)
4. Bacterial tracheitis
5. Simple URI
6. Subglottic hemangioma
7. Diphtheria

RULE OUT

The most important rule out considerations with cough are due to upper or lower airway obstruction such as peritonsillar or retropharyngeal abscess or epiglottitis. Important causes of lower airway obstruction include pneumonia, asthma, or inhaled foreign body.

VII. Diagnostic Findings

A. Laboratory Studies

1. Bronchitis

a. Leukocytosis
b. Sputum culture and Gram stain
c. Viral titers
d. Mycoplasma titers

2. Common Cold

a. Complete blood cell count (CBC) if symptoms persist for > 10 days or with temperature > 100 °F (37.8 °C).
b. Nasal smear for eosinophilia for patients in whom allergy is suspected.

3. Laryngotracheobronchitis

a. Leukopenia, early stage
b. Leukocytosis, severe later stage

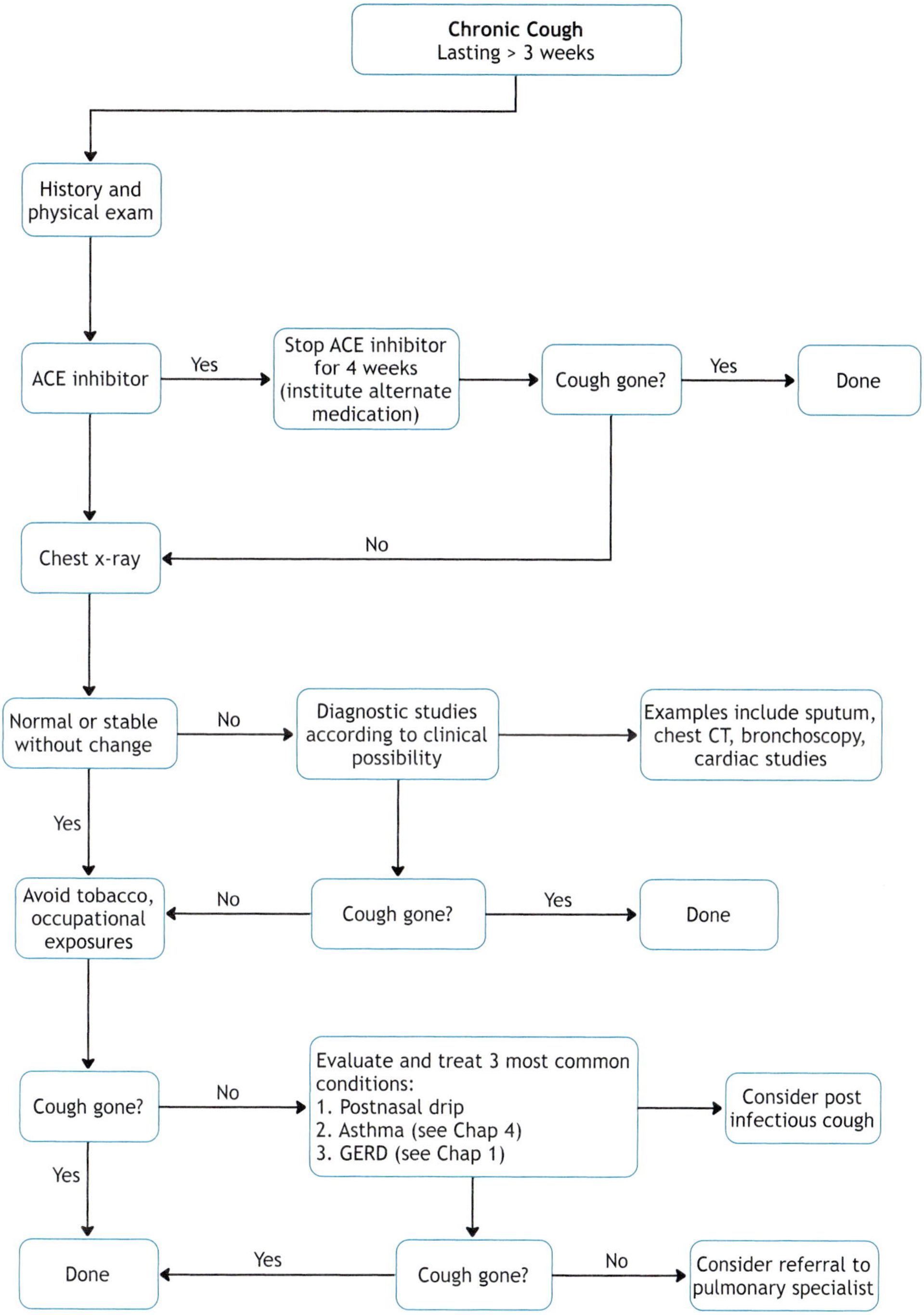

Figure 8–1 Evaluation of chronic cough in adults.

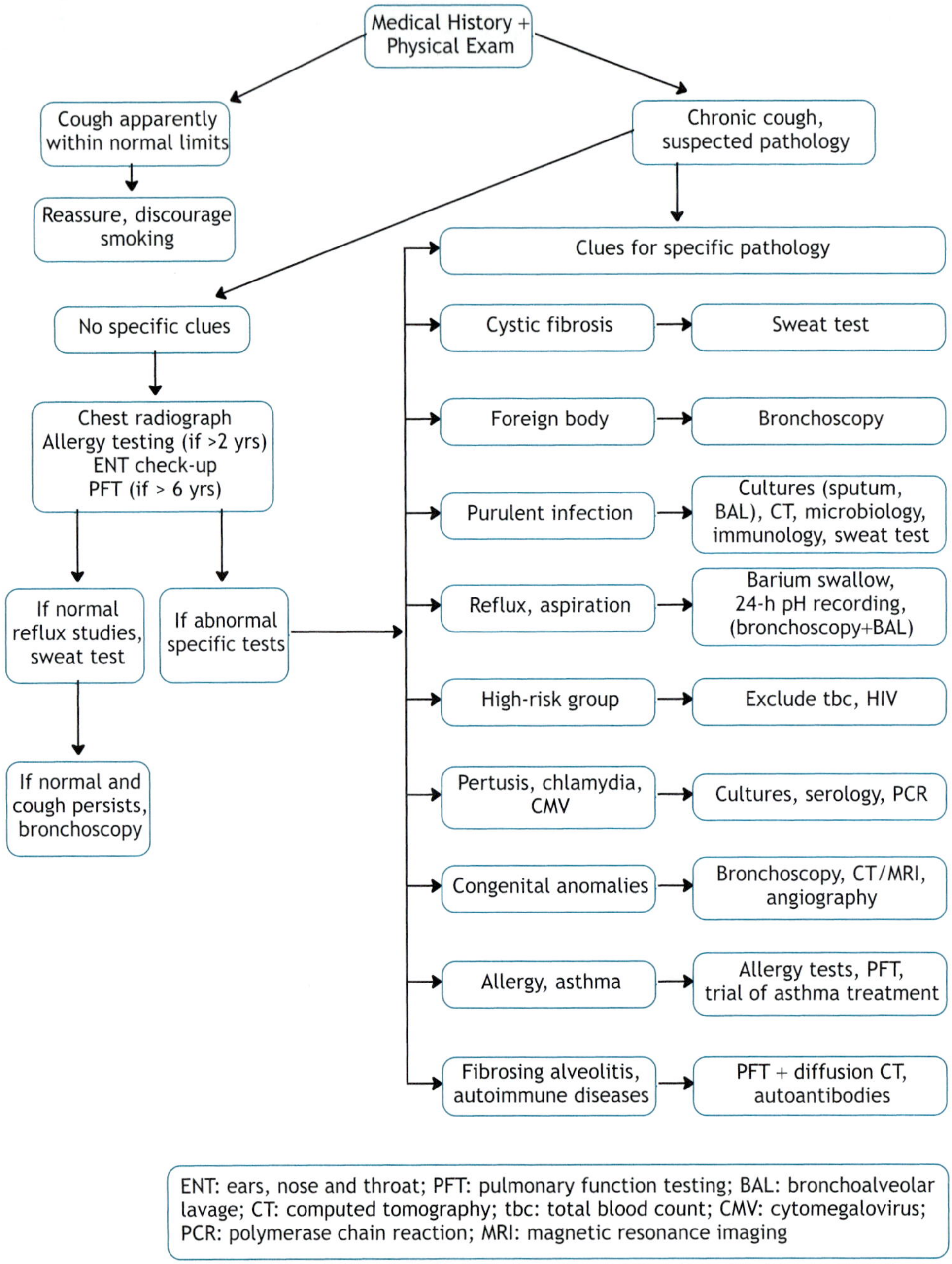

Figure 8–2 Evaluation of chronic cough in children.

B. Imaging Studies

1. **Bronchitis:** Chest x-ray reveals normal lungs if it is an uncomplicated case. Chest x-ray can help rule out other diseases if there is suspicion of other diseases.
2. **Common cold:** Imaging studies are unnecessary unless there is a concern that there is a bacterial superinfection of the sinuses, supraglottic region, trachea, or lungs.
3. **Laryngotracheobronchitis**
   a. **PA and lateral neck films** show funnel-shaped subglottic region with normal epiglottis (present in 40% of children with LTB).
   b. Patient should be monitored during imaging because progression of airway obstruction may be rapid.
4. **Chronic Cough**
   a. Chest x-ray
   b. Chest CT, if needed
   c. Upper gastrointestinal series
   d. Sinus series or sinus CT

C. Diagnostic Procedures

1. **Common cold:** In rare cases, it may be beneficial to attempt to culture virus from nasal washings or identify by ELISA or RIA methods.
2. **Laryngotracheobronchitis**
   a. Direct laryngoscopy, if the child is not in acute distress.
   b. Fiberoptic laryngoscopy, procedure of choice where available.
   c. Bronchoscopy
3. **Chronic cough** (see Figures 8–1 and 8–2)
   a. 24-hour pH probe
   b. Bronchoscopy, rarely
   c. Extensive testing only if indicated by the history and physical examination. Simple testing (chest x-ray, sinus studies) followed by empiric therapy is directed at likely underlying etiology.

VIII. Treatment (see Figures 8–1 and 8–2)

A. Bronchitis

1. Recommend rest until fever subsides.
2. Use steam inhalations and vaporizers.
3. Prescribe antibiotics, if bacterial etiology is suspected (eg, smokers).
4. Provide adequate hydration.
5. Stop smoking.
6. Treat associated illnesses (eg, GERD).
7. Use antitussive agents.
8. Increase fluids (up to 2–4 L/day) while febrile.
9. **Pharmacotherapy**
   a. **Amantadine or rimantadine,** if influenza A is suspected and is most effective if taken within 24–48 hours of development of symptoms.
   b. **Decongestants,** if bronchitis is accompanied by sinusitis.
   c. **Antipyretic analgesics** (eg, acetaminophen or ibuprofen) are a safe and effective way of reducing fever and treating any associated discomfort.

d. **Antibiotics** for more severe symptoms, including persistent high fever, concomitant chronic obstructive pulmonary disease (COPD), and purulent discharge.
   (1) Amoxicillin 500 mg q 8 h or trimethoprim-sulfamethoxazole DS q 12 h for routine infection.
   (2) Macrolide-clarithromycin 500 mg q 12 h or azithromycin for penicillin or sulfa allergy or mycoplasma infection.
   (3) Doxycycline 100 mg qd for 10 days if *Moraxella, Chlamydia,* or *Mycoplasma* infection is suspected.
   (4) Quinolone-levofloxacin 500 mg qd for more serious infection or if patient has not responded to another, previously prescribed antibiotic.

e. **Cough suppressant** for troublesome cough (do not prescribe to patients who have COPD); guaifenesin with codeine or dextromethorphan may be useful.

f. **Bronchodilators** (aerosols inhalants/steroids) are helpful for the reactive airway component.

g. Consider **steroids** for severe bronchospasm.

B. Common Cold

1. Recommend rest, fluids, and symptomatic measures.
2. Reassure that usual course of cold is 6–10 days.
3. Humidify inspired air.
4. Discontinue use of tobacco and alcohol products.
5. In infants, clear nasal passages with a bulb syringe, position mattress at 45°, and use saline nasal drops.
6. **Pharmacotherapy:** There are no medications that can cure the common cold, but some that target a particular symptom can reduce the likelihood of adverse systemic effects.
   a. **Topical decongestants** (sympathomimetics such as oxymetazoline) reduce edema and swelling of the nasal mucosa, promote drainage, and reduce nasal airflow resistance. These agents are preferred rather than oral agents because of minimal systemic effects. In children aged 6 and younger, nasal sprays are preferred over drops.
   b. **Topical anticholinergics** (eg, ipratropium) control rhinorrhea but do not relieve nasal congestion or sneezing.
   c. **Oral decongestants** (eg, pseudoephedrine) have a longer duration of action than do topical decongestants. There is also a lack of local irritation and no risk of rhinitis medicamentosa.
   d. **Antihistamines** (eg, chlorpheniramine or non-sedating antihistamines) are a safe and effective way to alleviate sneezing and rhinorrhea. Their benefit may be from anticholinergic effects, drying nasal and pharyngeal secretions, and sedative effects that promote rest.
   e. **Cough suppressants** (eg, codeine or dextromethorphan) are useful if a cough is nonproductive or interferes with sleep or normal activities.
   f. **Expectorants** (eg, guaifenesin) are commonly used but efficacy has not been proven.

C. Laryngotracheobronchitis

1. Feed frequently and increase fluids for mild cases.
2. In severe cases, patient may require IV fluids.

3. **Medications**
   a. **Dexamethasone** 0.6 mg/kg/day
   b. **Racemic epinephrine** 0.2–0.5 mL 2.25% racemic epinephrine delivered in 2–3 mL normal saline, 1 dose every 30 minutes. Monitor for side effects and rebound.
   c. Antibiotics are controversial for the treatment of this viral illness.
   d. Give **oxygen as needed.**

D. **Chronic Cough**
1. Direct treatment at most likely etiology.
2. **Eliminate smoking and angiotensin-converting enzyme (ACE) inhibitors.**
3. Offer empiric treatment for postnasal drip and GERD.
4. Attempt **maximal therapy** for single most likely cause for several weeks; if no improvement is shown, search for coexisting etiologies.
5. **Pharmacotherapy**
   a. **Antitussives**
      (1) **Dextromethorphan** 30 mg bid, age > 6 years
      (2) **Narcotics: codeine** 15–30 mg q 6 h, hydrocodone 5 mg q 6 h
   b. **Other treatments,** including antacids, bronchodilators, and antibiotics directed at etiology of cough

IX. Summary Table

Condition	Pathophysiology	Diagnostic Studies	Treatment
Viral URI	Viral infection	None	None or OTCs
Upper airway obstruction (peritonsillar abscess)	Bacterial infection, foreign body	CBC, culture	Antibiotics or bronchoscopic removal
Lower airway obstruction (pneumonia)	Bacterial infection	CBC, CXR	Antibiotics
Asthma	Airway inflammation and obstruction	None	Inhaled anti-inflammatory, bronchodilator
COPD	Alveolar disease	CXR, PFTs	Bronchodilator, oxygen
GERD	Acid reflux and possible aspiration	EGD or pH testing	Anti-reflux medication
Reactive airways disease	Airway inflammation	None	Bronchodilator
Bronchogenic carcinoma	Neoplastic	CXR, CT scan chest	As indicated by pathology

CBC, complete blood cell count; COPD, chronic obstructive pulmonary disease; CXR, chest x-ray; EGD, esophagogastroduodenoscopy; GERD, gastroesophageal reflux disease; OTC, over the counter; PFT, pulmonary function test; URI, upper respiratory infection.

CLINICAL CASE

A 10-year-old boy comes to the office with his mother because the boy has had a cough, sore throat, runny nose, and a temperature of 100.5 °F (38.1 ° C) for the past 3 days. The boy's mother says that he has had a dry, occasionally hacking cough but that he does not seem to bring anything up when he coughs. Two days ago, he complained of a sore throat and runny nose. His throat hurts but has not limited him from swallowing. The mother says that the boy's throat looks red at the back. His runny nose is characterized as a discharge that is slightly yellow and occasionally green. His temperature has been up and down, but no higher than 100.5 °F (38.1 °C). He is an otherwise well child who does well in school. He usually plays sports after school with his friends, but over the past few days he has been limited by the cough and sore throat. His mother is mainly worried because the cough has not gone away and the discharge from his nose looks green now. She thinks he would get better if he had some antibiotics. She says a lot of the children at school have been sick and their mothers say that they improved when given antibiotics. This boy's past history is otherwise normal. He has a few colds each year. He has never been hospitalized. He has received all of his immunizations. On physical examination, he appears non-toxic, although he is coughing in the examination room. His vital signs are all normal, including a pulse oximetry of 95%. HEENT examination demonstrates normal tympanic membranes and a red throat without exudates. The tonsils are not enlarged, and there is no cervical adenopathy. Chest examination reveals coarse upper respiratory sounds but no wheezes or crackles. Cardiovascular examination is normal as is the remainder of his physical examination.

Although this child presents with a very common and likely benign illness, **the challenge for the physician is to differentiate the majority of children with benign viral illnesses from the few with more serious diseases.** Secondarily, the physician is called upon to offer patient education and discuss antibiotic usage with a parent who thinks her child would benefit from these drugs.

Symptoms of a more serious illness could point to an upper or lower airway obstruction or to a severe headache. Upper airway obstruction could indicate a peritonsillar or retropharyngeal abscess or epiglottitis. Children with this condition may have a combination of high fever, severe sore throat with dysphagia, muffled voice, trismus, drooling, stridor, and medial deviation of the soft palate. These children need immediate triage, including consultation with an ear, nose, and throat specialist and/or emergency department management.

Lower airway obstruction could indicate pneumonia, asthma, or obstruction with a foreign body. These patients present with a combination of high fever, wheezing, and dyspnea. Physical examination would reveal wheezing and crackles as well as stridor if it were a foreign body. A severe headache could indicate a subarachnoid hemorrhage as a complication of sinusitis that eroded through the cribriform plate.

Our patient most likely has a viral URI, a self-limited illness that typically lasts from 5 to 14 days. Patients will report some combination of sore throat, rhinorrhea, cough, fever < 102 °F (38.9 °C) lasting < 3 days, and laryngitis. The onset of symptoms is rapid, with symptoms becoming worse during the first 3 to 5 days and then gradually beginning to improve. These symptoms will generally resolve within 7 to 14 days regardless of what is done. Patients can continue with a mild cough for up to 3 days after other symptoms resolve. The sinus discharge often begins as a clear liquid and changes to yellow; however, this does not indicate that a bacterial infection is present.

With this self-limiting viral illness, one of the most important roles for the physician is patient education. **Antibiotics are only effective for treating bacterial infections,** and they do not shorten the course or cure a patient with a viral illness. Unnecessary use of antibiotics will lead to the development of antibiotic-resistant strains of bacteria. However, many patients have the misconception that antibiotics will help shorten the illness or lead to symptom resolution more quickly.

Various over-the-counter preparations may lessen symptoms. Patients whose cough continues after the resolution of the illness may benefit from inhaled bronchodilators for the reactive airways disease. Some patients may also ask about the use of **herbal preparations,** including echinacea. Although current findings do not support the use of echinacea in preventing viral URIs, some data suggest that it may shorten the course of URIs. It is important for the physician to remain current with the literature.

The work-up of our patient, who we believe has a viral upper respiratory infection, is limited. If there were concerns about bronchitis, laryngotracheobronchitis, or a bacterial infection, the work-up would be more extensive.

CLINICAL PEARLS

Most cases of cough are benign and self-limiting and antibiotics are not helpful.

CHAPTER 9
DEPRESSION

I. Defining Features

A. **Depressed moods** can vary from mild sadness to intense feelings of guilt, worthlessness, and hopelessness.

B. **Cognitive problems** can include difficulties in concentration, ruminations, and a lack of decisiveness.

C. **Loss of interest** can be seen as decreased involvement in daily activities (ie, work and recreation).

D. **Somatic complaints** include headache; disrupted, lessened, or excessive sleep; loss of energy; change in appetite; and decreased sex drive.

E. Anxiety and/or irritability are often present.

II. Epidemiology

A. In the United States, the **incidence of major depression among the population is 17%.**

B. Approximately 10% of the population suffers from depression in any 12-month period.

C. **An estimated 5–20% of the population will experience a significant depressive episode at some time.**

D. As many as 50% of depressed patients may not be correctly diagnosed.

E. The mean age at diagnosis of bipolar disorder (manic depressive disorder) is age 30, and the mean age for unipolar disorder (depressive disorder) is age 40.

F. **Depression is more common in females than in males.**

G. About 50% of patients who have a depressive episode will have another episode within 2 years.

H. **Untreated depression can lead to suicide.**

I. Men usually are successful in committing suicide; however, women attempt suicide more often but have a lower mortality rate.

J. **Patients who have depression have a lifetime risk of suicide of 10–15%.**

III. Pathophysiology

A. Depression is associated with **dysfunction of the receptor-neurotransmitter** relationship in the **limbic system.**

B. **Serotonin and norepinephrine** are the primary neurotransmitters involved, but dopamine also has been implicated in depression.

C. There is strong epidemiologic evidence of a **genetic contribution,** especially for **bipolar disorders,** and **heritability is estimated to be as high as 80%.** The influence of genes in major unipolar depression is less clear than for bipolar disorder.

D. In **unipolar depression,** the candidate genes that demonstrate the greatest promise belong to the serotonergic system: tyrosine hydroxylase, the serotonin (5-hydroxytryptamine [5-HT]) transporter, and the 5-HT2C receptor.

E. **Depression** is a complex disorder in which several genes of modest effect interact with each other or with a variety of environmental factors to increase **familial susceptibility for the disorder.**

IV. Risk Factors

A. **Age:** Adolescence, menopause, retirement, advancing age

B. **Economic conditions:** Stressful situations

C. **Bereavement:** Insomnia, losses

D. **Social relationships:** Children with behavioral disorders, especially hyperactivity; substance abuse; strong family history of depression, suicide, alcoholism, or other substance abuse.

E. **Physical health:** Chronic disease (especially multiple coexisting diseases); migraine headaches; back pain; chronic pain; recent myocardial infarction; peptic ulcer disease.

F. **Postpartum period:** Up to 80% of women experience some mild letdown of mood within 6 months after giving birth.

V. Clinical Presentation

A. **Symptoms of depression:** The *Diagnostic and Statistical Manual of Mental Disorders,* 4th edition, Text Revision (DSM-IV-TR), criteria are used to determine the diagnosis of depression (Table 9–1). The patient must have a total of 5 of the listed symptoms for at least 2 weeks, and 1 of the symptoms must be depressed mood or loss of interest. Another approach suggests that depression is probable when at least 4 of the following common symptoms exist, in addition to depressed mood or anhedonia:

1. **Poor appetite:** Either weight gain or weight loss
2. **Sleep disorder:** Either insomnia or hypersomnia
3. **Fatigue:** Out of proportion to the amount of energy expended
4. **Psychomotor retardation or agitation:** Restlessness, irritability, or withdrawal
5. **Poor self-image:** Self-reproach, excessive guilt
6. **Cognitive problems:** Difficulty concentrating, poor memory, unable to make decisions
7. **Suicidal ideation:** Sometimes when people begin to recover from depression, they gain enough energy to think about and attempt suicide.

B. **Signs of depression:** There are no specific physical examination findings in depression.

Table 9–1. DSM-IV-TR criteria used in the diagnosis of depression.

Patient must have a total of 5 symptoms for at least 2 weeks. One of the symptoms must be depressed mood or loss of interest.
1. Depressed mood (as indicated either in a subjective report or observation made by others)
2. Markedly diminished interest or pleasure in all or almost all activities (as indicated either in a subjective report or observation made by others)
3. Significant (> 5% body weight) weight loss or gain or increase or decrease in appetite
4. Insomnia or hypersomnia
5. Psychomotor agitation or retardation (observable by others, not merely subjective feelings of restlessness or being slowed down)
6. Fatigue or loss of energy nearly every day
7. Feeling of worthlessness or inappropriate guilt (which may be delusional) nearly every day (not merely self-reproach or guilt about being sick)
8. Diminished concentration or indecisiveness nearly every day (either by subjective account or as observed by others)
9. Recurrent thoughts of death (not just fear of dying), recurrent suicidal ideation without a specific plan, or a suicide attempt or a specific plan for committing suicide

CLINICAL SKILLS TIP

Depression is a clinical diagnosis based predominately on patient history. Screening instruments such as SIGECAPS are very helpful in determining a diagnosis (Table 9–2).

VI. Differential Diagnosis (Figure 9–1)

A. **Medical conditions:** Organic brain diseases; diabetes mellitus; endocrine diseases such as hypothyroid and hyperthyroid diseases; liver failure; renal failure; chronic fatigue syndrome; vitamin deficiency (pernicious anemia, pellagra); side effects of medication (many drugs cause or worsen depression); medication overdose and/or abuse.

B. **Substance use and abuse:** Withdrawal from medication; alcohol abuse; substance abuse; withdrawal from abused substance (alcohol, cocaine, marijuana).

C. **Bereavement:** Attention must be given to personal life adjustment problems and the roles of medication, because depression can be associated as a part of any illness, either reactively or as a secondary symptom.

Table 9–2. SIGECAPS.

To meet the diagnosis of major depression, a patient must have 4 of the following symptoms plus depressed mood or anhedonia for at least 2 weeks. To meet the diagnosis of dysthymic disorder, a patient must have 2 of the following 6 symptoms marked with an asterisk, plus depression for at least 2 years.
Sleep disorder (either increased or decreased sleep)*
Interests deficit (anhedonia)
Guilt (worthlessness,* hopelessness,* regret)
Energy deficit*
Concentration deficit*
Appetite (either decreased or increased)*
Psychomotor agitation or slowing
Suicidal ideation

RULE OUT

It is important to rule out substance abuse. Use the CAGE questions when evaluating the patient (Table 9–3).

VII. Diagnostic Findings

A. **Imaging Studies:** If organic brain syndrome is suspected, a CT scan or MRI of the brain can be performed.

B. **Diagnostic Procedures**

1. Depression is primarily a clinical diagnosis that depends on skillfully eliciting information about family, social, and psychosocial factors.
2. To assist in identifying and following depressed patients, validated standard rating scales can be used.
   a. **SIGECAPS** (see Table 9–2)
   b. Zung Self-rating Depression Scale (STS)
   c. Beck Depression Inventory (BDI)
   d. Criteria for Epidemiologic Studies Depression Scale (CES-D)
   e. Children's Depression Inventory (CDI)
   f. Yesavage Geriatric Depression Scale
3. An **electrocardiogram** (ECG) can be used to diagnose arrhythmia (especially heart block).
4. An **electroencephalogram** (EEG) may be performed if organic brain disease is suspected.

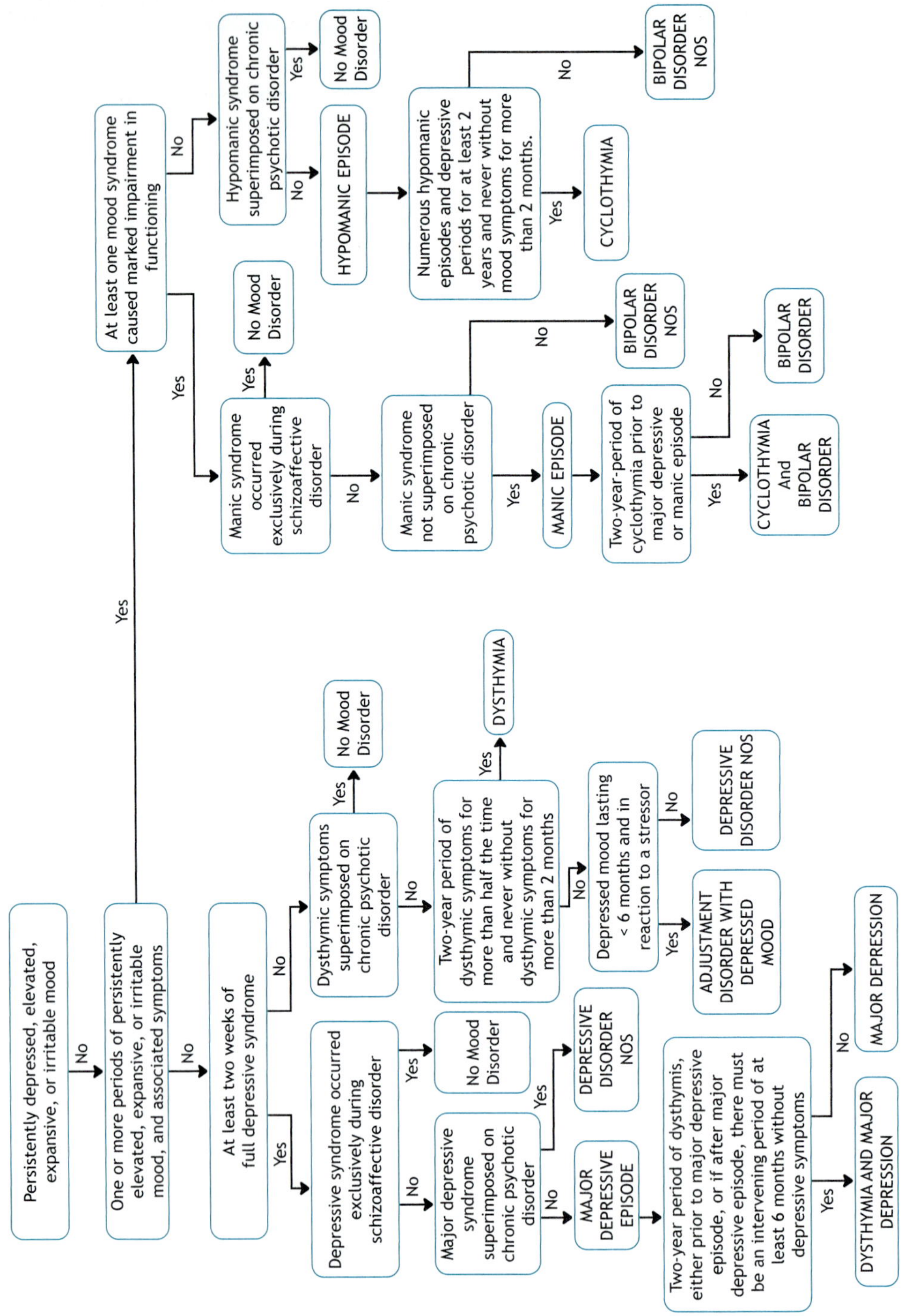

Figure 9–1 Decision tree for the differential diagnosis of mood disturbances.

Table 9–3. CAGE screening questions for alcoholism.

	Have you ever
C	Felt you ought to **cut** down on your drinking?
A	Had people **annoy** you by criticizing your drinking?
G	Felt bad or **guilty** about your drinking?
E	Had a drink as an **eye opener** first thing in the morning to steady your nerves or get rid of a hangover or to get the day started?

5. Depression is an underdiagnosed illness, often due to the masking and under-reporting of symptoms by patients.

VIII. Treatment (Figures 9–2 and 9–3)

A. In **depression associated with reactive disorders,** psychotherapy and the passage of time can be used without drug therapy.

B. **Cognitive-behavioral therapy** is the most effective treatment for **depression in children.** Individual therapy sessions have proved more effective than family sessions.

C. **Anti-depressant Drugs**

1. **Serotonin-selective reuptake inhibitors (SSRIs)**
   a. Fluoxetine
   b. Sertraline
   c. Paroxetine
   d. Fluvoxamine
   e. Citalopram
   f. Escitalopram
2. **Atypical anti-depressants**
   a. Bupropion
   b. Venlafaxine
   c. Nefazodone
   d. Mirtazapine
3. **Tricyclic antidepressants**
   a. Amitriptyline
   b. Clomipramine
   c. Imipramine
   d. Nortriptyline
   e. Desipramine
4. **Monoamine oxidase inhibitors (MAOIs):** MAOIs usually are used as third-line drugs in the treatment of depression because of dietary restrictions (foods high in tyramine such as cheese, wine, and salami). MAOIs can cause symptoms of sympathomimetic effects and central nervous system effects.

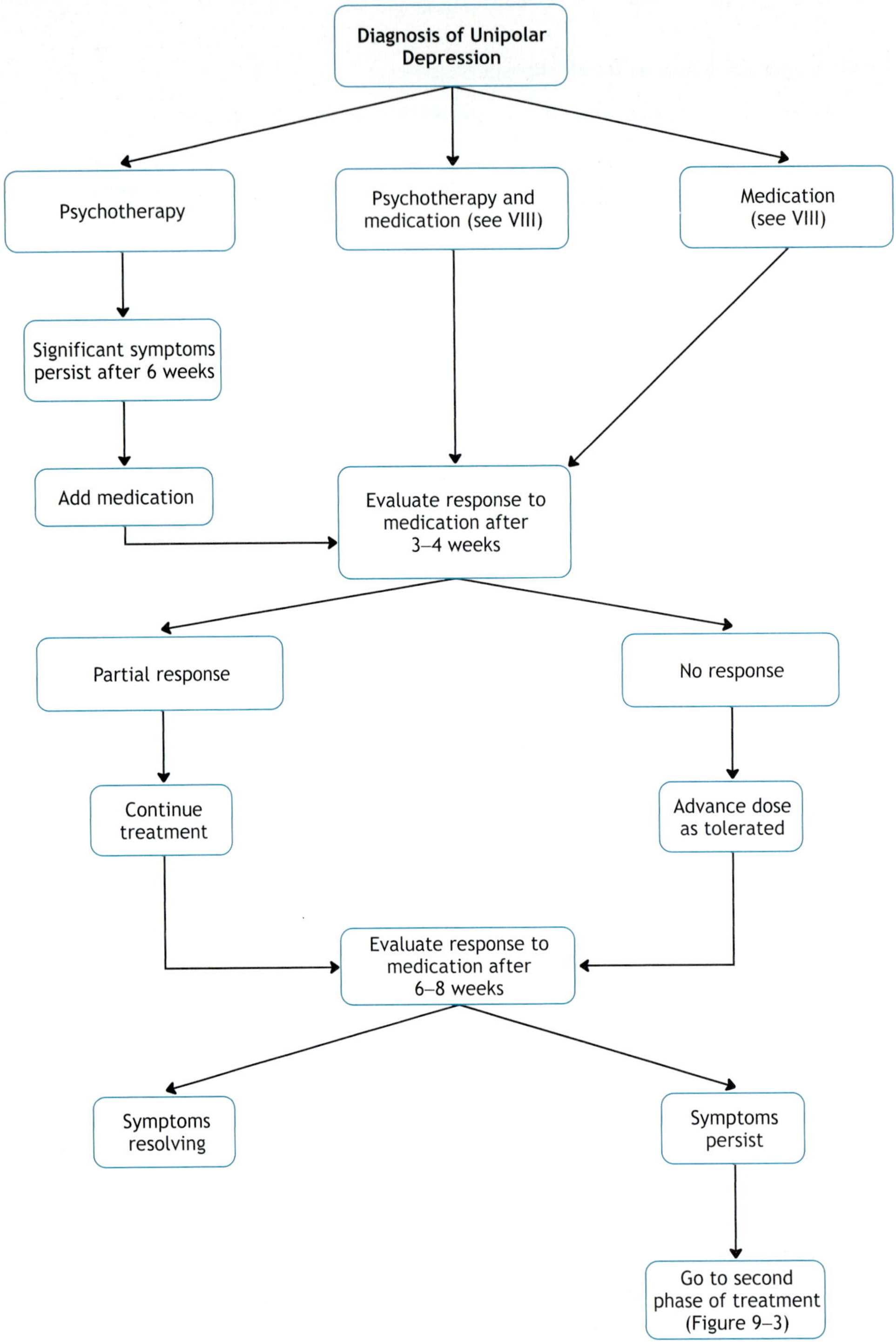

Figure 9–2 Initial phase of treatment for depression.

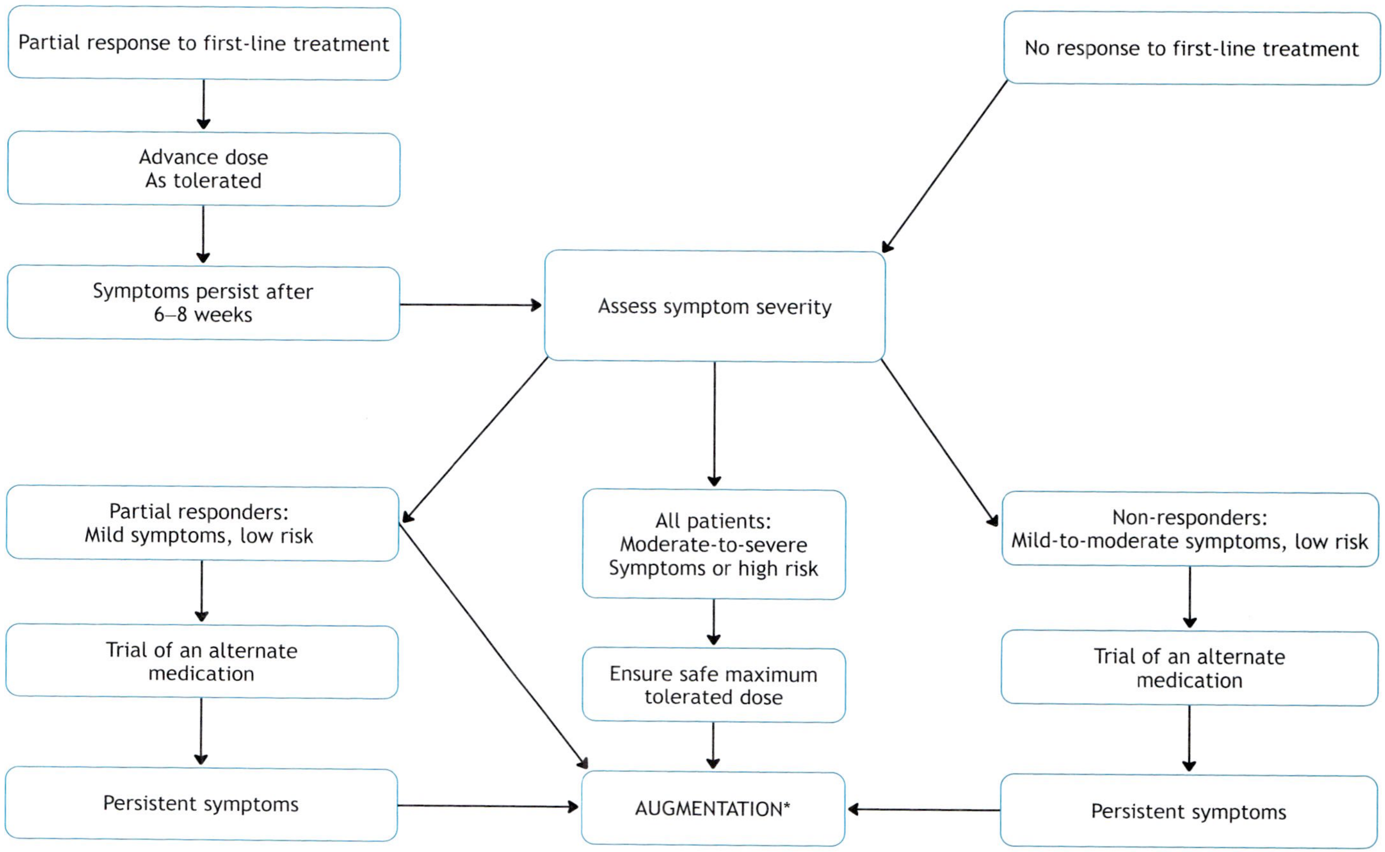

*Augmentation involves the use of a combination of medications to enhance the efficacy of an antidepressant

Figure 9–3 Second phase of treatment for depression.

IX. Summary Table

Condition	Pathophysiology	Diagnostic Studies	Treatment
Depression	Changes in receptor-neurotransmitter relationship in limbic system	Standardized questionnaire SIGECAPS or CAGE, thyroid function tests, CT scan or MRI of brain, if organic brain disease is suspected	Psychotherapy, antidepressant drugs
Organic brain disease	Unknown	CT scan or MRI of brain	
Hypothyroidism	Decrease in available thyroid hormone	Thyroid-stimulating hormone	Thyroid replacement
Chronic fatigue syndrome (CFS)	Unknown/multi-factorial	Blood chemistries and multiple other diagnostic studies (many other diseases must be ruled-out before arriving at diagnosis of CFS)	Multi-factorial
Side effects of medications	Medication-dependent	None	Withdraw drug or change drug or learn to tolerate the medication
Alcohol or other substance abuse	Related to substance	None	Withdrawal protocol
Withdrawal from abused substance	Related to substance	None	Withdrawal protocol

CT, computer tomography; MRI, magnetic resonance imagine.

CLINICAL CASE

A-48-year-old woman comes to see you at the urging of her family because they think that she seems to have lost interest in her usual activities and her family. The woman does not think this should be a major concern, but she does acknowledge that over the past month she has experienced markedly decreased interest in her regular activities. She cannot think of any particular inciting event, but she says that things just do not seem worthwhile and she has no energy to do all of the things she used to do, even though she says that she is sleeping about 10 hours every night. She also says that she cannot make decisions anymore, either at home or at work. Some things have gone wrong, and she feels totally responsible for them. She says that for about 2 weeks after the birth of both of her children she felt "down," but the feeling went away. She is sitting on the examination table with her head down. She denies having eating problems, and her weight has been stable. She has no chronic medical problems and takes no medications. She has never used tobacco, alcohol, or recreational drugs. She is a single parent. There are no concerns of domestic abuse or violence from the father of her children. On physical examination, her vital signs are within normal limits She responds to all questions asked, but initiates little discussion. She denies any history of psychiatric illness or of having suicidal thoughts. HEENT, cardiac, and pulmonary examinations are within normal limits. There is no thyromegaly, and the neurologic examination is also within normal limits.

On first walking into the room, you notice that the patient appears depressed. Her head is down and her face is without expression. As we know, our examination begins as we open the door to see the patient. If these first clinical impressions are validated through the history and physical examination, they are extremely valuable. Fortunately, there are objective guidelines to help us in the evaluation of a patient who appears depressed.

The first guideline is from the DSM-IV-TR definition of major depression (see Table 9–1). To begin an interview in which you suspect depression, ask the patient the following questions:

Over the past month have you been bothered by

1. Loss of interest or pleasure in daily activities?
2. Feeling down, depressed, or hopeless?

If either of these diagnostic findings is positive, you can then **pursue the diagnosis using other structured questionnaires and instruments** (see VII B). One set of questions found to be extremely helpful in the primary care setting is using the mnemonic **SIGECAPS** (see Table 9–2).

Although this patient's presentation was quite straightforward, you (the physician) must look for comorbid diseases and other explanations for the patient's symptoms. Thyroid disease can cause some of these symptoms. A direct physiologic effect of a substance (eg, a drug of abuse or a medication such as reserpine, steroids, alphamethyldopa, propranolol, and some hormonal therapies) can also account for these symptoms. **It is also important to consider bipolar disorder.** Questions might include the following:

Has there been a distinct period of abnormally and persistently elevated, expansive, or irritable mood, lasting at least 1 week?

During the period of mood disturbance, have 3 (or more) of the following symptoms persisted (4 if the mood is only irritable) and have they been present to a significant degree?

1. Inflated self-esteem or grandiosity
2. Decreased need for sleep
3. More talkative than usual or pressure to keep talking
4. Flight of ideas or subjective experience that thoughts are racing
5. Distractibility
6. Increase in goal-directed activity or psychomotor agitation
7. Excessive involvement in pleasurable activities that have a high potential for painful consequences

If these criteria are met, the patient may have a bipolar mood disorder. This is particularly important to identify because treatment for this disorder differs from other disorders.

It is important to determine if substance abuse is present. A commonly used screening tool is the **CAGE-AID questionnaire.** Before using that questionnaire, these 2 questions should be asked:

1. Do you drink alcohol?
2. Have you experimented with drugs?

If the patient acknowledges experimenting with drugs, ask the CAGE-AID questions. CAGE-AID questions are modified from the CAGE, as noted by *italicized* text.

CAGE-AID QUESTIONNAIRE

Have you ever

C felt you ought to **cut** down on your drinking (*or drug use*)?

A had people **annoy** you by criticizing your drinking (*or drug use*)?

G felt bad or **guilty** about your drinking (*or drug use*)?

E had a drink (*or used drugs*) as an **eye opener** first thing in the morning to steady your nerves or get rid of a hangover or to get the day started?

The primary objective in using any standardized questionnaire is that it will quantify and document future progress, including response and remission rates.

The most important triage issue in primary care is to assess suicide risk, which is often difficult to do with depressed patients. Consider asking the following questions:

1. Do you feel that life is not worth living?
2. Do you wish you were dead?
3. Have you thought about ending your life?
4. If yes, have you gone so far as to think about how you would do so?
5. Do you have access to a way to carry out your plan?
6. What keeps you from harming yourself?

When there is risk of suicide, you must contact a mental health professional and consider emergent psychiatric hospitalization.

In the absence of suicide risk or need for emergent hospitalization, the physician must design a treatment plan, which will likely include psychotherapy, pharmacotherapy, and a follow-up plan. Adherence to a therapeutic drug dose and meeting clinical goals are more important than the specific antidepressant chosen. Depression is associated with changes in the receptor-neurotransmitter relationship in the limbic system (see III). The currently available antidepressants will work in this axis. The available classes of antidepressants are listed in section VIII. The **choice of antidepressant should be based on**

1. The patient's history of response to a previously prescribed antidepressant drug, if there is a history.
2. The patient's comorbid psychiatric or medical conditions.
3. The physician's familiarity with specific antidepressant drugs.

CLINICAL PEARLS

Depression is an under-diagnosed illness. The family physician must suspect the disease and use standardized instruments, such as SIGECAPS, to determine the correct diagnosis.

CHAPTER 10
DIABETES MELLITUS TYPE 1

I. Defining Features

A. After an overnight fast, plasma glucose is ≥ 126 mg/dL. This level must be documented on more than 1 occasion.

B. The 2-h postload glucose is ≥ 200 mg/dL during an oral glucose tolerance test (OGTT). The test should be performed using a glucose load containing the equivalent of 75 g anhydrous glucose dissolved in water.

C. In the absence of unequivocal hyperglycemia, these criteria should be confirmed by repeat testing on a different occasion. The OGTT is not recommended for routine clinical use.

D. Ketonemia or ketonuria, or both, are present.

E. Islet autoantibodies are frequently present.

F. Random plasma glucose ≥ 200 mg/dL is associated with polyuria, polydipsia, and/or weight loss.

II. Epidemiology

A. The **lifetime risk** of diabetes mellitus (DM) is **10% in the western hemisphere.**

B. The United States has an **average incidence** of 0.015% (15/100,000), with higher incidences in states more densely populated with persons of Scandinavian descent such as Minnesota. An estimated 3 of 1000 persons develop type 1 DM by age 20 years.

C. About **1.4 million people in the United States have type 1 DM.**

D. **Caucasians have the highest reported incidence of type 1 DM; Chinese have the lowest.**

E. Type 1 DM is 1.5 times more likely to develop in American whites than in American blacks or Hispanics.

F. The **mean age of onset of type 1 DM is between 8 and 12 years old,** with a peak during adolescence. A rapid decline in incidence occurs after adolescence.

G. Onset is about 1.5 years earlier in girls than in boys.

H. Monozygotic twins have a 60% lifetime concordance for developing type 1 DM, although only 30% do so within 10 years after the first twin is diagnosed.

In contrast, dizygotic twins have only an 8% risk of concordance, which is similar to the risk among other siblings.

I. HLA class II molecules DR3 and DR4 are associated strongly with type 1 DM. More than 90% of whites with type 1 DM express 1 or both of these molecules, compared with 50–60% in the general population. The expression of both DR3 and DR4 carries the greatest risk of type 1 DM; these patients have characteristics of both the DR3 and DR4 groups.

J. **Complications** of diabetes include retinopathy, neuropathy, nephropathy, heart disease, and stroke.

III. Pathophysiology

A. **Type 1 DM** is a **chronic** disease caused by **pancreatic insufficiency (deficiency) of insulin production,** resulting in hyperglycemia and end-organ complications such as accelerated atherosclerosis, neuropathy, nephropathy, and retinopathy.

B. **Immune-mediated type 1 DM** is thought to result from an infectious or toxic insult to patients whose immune systems are genetically predisposed to develop a vigorous autoimmune response either against altered pancreatic beta-cell antigens or against molecules of the beta cell resembling the viral protein (molecular mimicry).

C. **Idiopathic type 1 DM** is the diagnosis given to those patients who have no evidence of pancreatic beta cell autoimmunity to explain their insulinopenia and ketoacidosis. This subgroup is comprised of < 10% of patients with type 1 DM and is **called type 1B.**

IV. Risk Factors

A. About **95% of patients with type 1 DM possess either the gene HLA-DR3 or HLA-DR4,** compared with 45–50% of Caucasian controls.

B. HLA-DQ genes are more specific markers of type 1 susceptibility, since a particular variety (HLA-DQB1*0302) is found in the HLA-DR4 patients with type 1 DM, while a "protective" gene (HLA-DQB1*0602) is often present in the HLA-DR4 controls.

C. Most patients with type 1 DM at diagnosis have circulating antibodies to islet cell antibodies (ICA), to insulin (IAA), to glutamic acid decarboxylase (GAD 65), and to tyrosine phosphatases (IA-2 and IA2-β).

D. Patients who carry **either the HLA-DR3 or the HLA-DR4 gene** have an increased **risk factor of 4.** Patients who carry **both susceptibility genes** have an increased relative **risk factor of 12.**

E. Patients who carry HLA-B8 and HLA-B15 genes also have a higher risk.

F. If a mother or father has type 1 DM, the child has a greater risk of developing DM.

G. **There is a greater risk of developing DM if any first-degree relative has either type 1 or type 2 DM.**

V. Clinical Presentation

A. **Symptoms**

1. Polyuria, polydipsia, polyphagia

2. Anorexia (commonly observed)
3. Weight loss (usually from 10–30%, and often almost devoid of body fat at time of diagnosis)
4. Increased fatigue
5. Muscle cramps
6. Irritability and emotional lability
7. Vision changes, such as blurriness
8. Altered school and work performance
9. Chest pain and occasional difficulty breathing
10. Abdominal discomfort and pain
11. Nausea, diarrhea, or constipation

B. **Signs are limited unless the patient presents with ketoacidosis.**
1. Fruity (ketone) odor of breath
2. Abnormal breathing pattern (deep, rapid respirations often called Kussmaul breathing, due to acidosis)

CLINICAL SKILLS TIP

Polyuria, polydipsia, and polyphagia are classic presenting symptoms in a patient with type 1 DM. When these symptoms are accompanied by fatigue and weight loss, the physician should suspect and test for diabetes.

VI. Differential Diagnosis

A. Benign renal glycosuria

B. Glucose intolerance

C. Type 2 DM. (Children may have maturity onset diabetes of the young [MODY], which is becoming more frequent.)

D. Infantile-onset diabetes mellitus

E. **Secondary diabetes**
1. Pancreatic disease (pancreatitis, cystic fibrosis)
2. Hormonal disorders (pheochromocytoma, multiple endocrine adenomatosis)
3. Inborn errors of metabolism (glycogen storage disease type I)
4. Genetic disorders with insulin resistance (acanthosis nigricans)
5. Drug- or chemical-induced glucose intolerance
6. Acute poisonings
   a. Salicylate poisoning can be associated with hyperglycemia and glycosuria.
   b. It may mimic diabetic ketoacidosis.

RULE OUT

Although there are multiple diagnoses in the differential, the physician must rule out type 1 DM before proceeding to investigate other diagnoses (see VI).

VII. Diagnostic Findings

A. **Laboratory Studies**
1. **Urinalysis**
   a. Glucosuria
   b. Ketonuria

2. **Blood testing procedures**
   a. **Glucose tolerance test**
      (1) **Methodology and normal fasting glucose:** Plasma and serum from venous blood samples has the advantage over whole blood of providing glucose values that are independent of hematocrit and that reflect the glucose concentration to which body tissues are exposed.
      (2) **Criteria for laboratory confirmation of DM:** If the fasting plasma glucose level is > 126 mg/dL on 1 or more occasions, further evaluation of the patient using a glucose challenge is unnecessary. If the fasting plasma glucose is < 126 mg/dL in suspected cases, a standardized OGTT may be performed (Table 10–1).
   b. **Serum fructosamine**
   c. **Ongoing management and monitoring tests**
      (1) **Glycated hemoglobin (hemoglobin A_1) measurements:** Glycated hemoglobin is abnormally high in diabetics who have chronic hyperglycemia and reflects their metabolic control. This measurement can be used to monitor a patient's blood glucose level over a 3-month period.
      (2) **Self-monitoring of blood glucose**
      (3) **Continuous glucose monitoring systems**
3. **Lipoprotein abnormalities in DM:** In type 1 DM, moderately deficient control of hyperglycemia is associated with only a slight elevation of LDL cholesterol and serum triglycerides and little if any change in HDL cholesterol.

VIII. Treatment (Figure 10–1)

A. **Types of Insulin**
   1. **Ultra-short-acting**
      a. Insulin lispro
      b. Insulin aspart
   2. **Short-acting**
      a. Regular Novolin
      b. Regular Humulin
   3. **Intermediate-acting**
      a. NPH Humulin
      b. NPH Novolin

Table 10–1. Criteria for oral glucose tolerance test (OGTT).

Oral Glucose Tolerance Test	Normal Glucose Tolerance	Impaired Glucose Tolerance	Diabetes Mellitus
Fasting plasma glucose	< 110 mg/dL	110–125 mg/dL	≥ 126 mg/dL
Two hours after glucose load	< 140 mg/dL	≥ 140 mg/dL but < 200 mg/dL	≥ 200 mg/dL

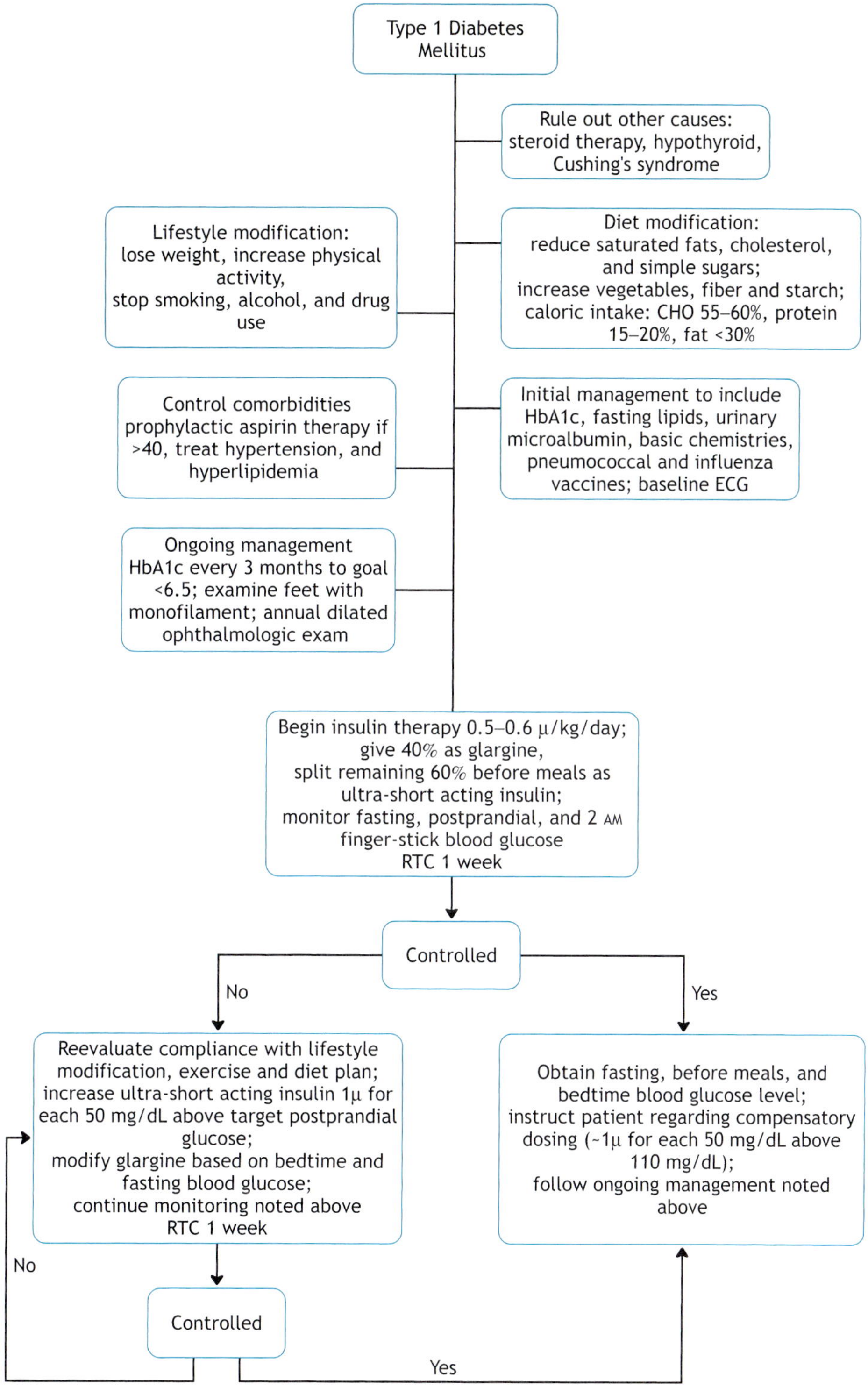

Figure 10–1 Treatment of the patient with type 1 diabetes mellitus.

4. **Premixed (%NPH/%regular)**
   a. Novolin 70/30
   b. Humulin 70/30
   c. Humalog mix 75/25 (%NPL/%insulin lispro)
5. **Long-acting**
   a. Insulin glargine
   b. Ultralente Humulin

B. Prevention of Complications

1. **Patients whose blood glucose levels are near normal** have a delayed onset and slowing of the progression of established microvascular and neuropathic complications of diabetes (diabetic neuropathy, nephropathy, and retinopathy).
2. Hypoglycemia can result from a delay in eating or unusual physical exertion.
3. Patients should carry packets of table sugar or candy at all times for use of onset of hypoglycemic symptoms. Patients' family and friends should be instructed on how to give an ampule of glucagon (1 mg) in the event that the patient is unconscious or refuses food.

IX. Summary Table

Disease	Pathophysiology	Diagnostic Studies	Treatment
Type I DM	Absolute insulinopenia	FBS or random blood glucose (OGTT rarely necessary)	Insulin
Type 2 DM	Insulin resistance	FBS and/or OGTT	Oral hypoglycemic agents, insulin, weight loss
Secondary diabetes due to cystic fibrosis	Insulinopenia (may not be absolute)	FBS and/or OGTT	Insulin
Urinary tract infection	Infectious	Urinalysis	Antibiotic

FBS, fasting blood sugar; OGTT, oral glucose tolerance test.

CLINICAL CASE

An 11-year-old-girl is brought by her mother to the emergency department because the child is confused and significantly dehydrated. The girl was in her usual state of good health until about 2 days ago when her mother noticed that she was drinking copious amounts of water and making hourly trips to the bathroom during the day and at night. The girl denies any problems with urination such as burning or foul smelling urine, but she does say that the urine seems almost like water. Normally, the girl is talkative, but she sits extremely quietly during the inter-

view and has a dazed look on her face. She does not respond to any questions, so her mother answers them for her. Although her appetite has been good, she has lost weight. Her mother had to dress her before coming to the emergency room because she was too confused. The girl's family history is unknown because she was adopted as a newborn. According to the mother, the girl is doing well in school and socially. She is not sexually active and uses no substances of abuse. Her physical examination shows elevated pulse and low blood pressure. She is breathing rapidly and deeply, and there is a fruity odor to her breath. Her weight is 6% below her last measured weight in the office 1 month ago. Her mucous membranes are extremely dry, and there is tenting of her skin. Her extremities are cool. Other than the findings related to her vital signs, no other abnormalities of her heart or lungs were found on examination. Her neurologic examination shows no focal deficit. She is able to follow commands, but responds very slowly.

This is an acute clinical scenario and needs to be addressed emergently. The child has moderately severe dehydration, and the fruity odor on her breath suggests **ketoacidosis.** The abnormal pattern of breathing (Kussmaul breathing) is characteristic of acidosis. Her vital signs of elevated pulse and low blood pressure are worrisome for hemodynamic instability. **A rapid diagnosis and initiation of treatment of this patient are necessary.**

Needing to urinate frequently could be due to a urinary tract infection. However, although she has polyuria, she is not experiencing dysuria or urgency. There is nothing to suggest any other infectious etiology (eg, cough, fever). Ingestion of a toxic substance must always be considered in a confused patient, although there is nothing to suggest drug use in this patient. Metabolic abnormalities must always be considered in an otherwise nonfocal history and physical examination. Although there are inflammatory conditions that could explain the mental status abnormalities, they are unlikely to present so acutely. This child most likely has type 1 DM and metabolic ketoacidosis.

Treatment should first aim to stabilize this patient hemodynamically with isotonic saline solution. The first set of diagnostic studies should include a urinalysis, finger stick blood glucose, and a metabolic profile. The urinalysis most likely would show an extremely dilute specific gravity, positive glucose and ketones, and no signs of infection. Her finger stick would show a range higher than the range of the glucose meter, and the metabolic profile would show hyperglycemia, hypokalemia, and acidosis (bicarbonate would be very low). Her serum sodium level may also be abnormally low at onset. **Management of this patient would continue with aggressive fluid resuscitation, short-acting insulin, and potassium.**

The child likely has a genetic predisposition to DM (although her family history is unknown) and either suffered an infectious or toxic insult (see III). Insulinopenia led to the inability of the cells to uptake and utilize glucose, which resulted in hyperglycemia.

Hyperglycemia was above the renal threshold, and glucose spilled into her urine. Glucosuria acts as an osmotic agent pulling water into the urine. This child demonstrates polyuria, compensatory polydipsia, and weight loss due to the cells' inability to utilize glucose. Potassium is leached from the cells and spilled into the urine. Without glucose, the cells begin to break down fatty acid, resulting in ketoacidosis. Although insulin and fluids can correct her hemodynamic and metabolic abnormalities, **type 1 DM is a chronic disease. Patients who have DM are at risk of multiple long-term sequelae** involving the eyes, kidneys, nervous system, and microvascular system.

CLINICAL PEARLS

Polyuria and polydipsia in the absence of infectious urinary tract symptoms, Kussmaul breathing, and the fruity odor of ketones on the patient's breath would lead the physician to a diagnosis of type 1 DM and ketoacidosis.

CHAPTER 11

DIABETES MELLITUS TYPE 2

I. Defining Features

A. **Most patients with type 2 diabetes mellitus (DM) are older than 40 years and are obese.**

B. **Polyuria and polydipsia** may be present. In women, **candidal vaginitis** may be an initial manifestation. Many patients are asymptomatic initially.

C. After an overnight fast, plasma glucose is ≥ 126 mg/dL and should be documented on more than 1 occasion. Two hours after drinking 75 g oral glucose, diagnostic values are ≥ 200 mg/dL.

D. Hypertension, dyslipidemia, and atherosclerosis are often associated conditions.

E. **Maturity onset diabetes of the young (MODY)** is characterized by a nonketotic type 2 DM inherited as an autosomal dominant mode, and appears in persons **younger than age 25.**

II. Epidemiology

A. In the United States, **over 90% of all patients with DM have type 2.**

B. The **incidence** of type 2 DM is **300/100,000** (men 230/100,000 and women 340/100,000).

C. The **prevalence is 5,000/100,000.**

D. Type 2 DM is more common in groups such as the Pima Indians.

E. In Caucasian populations, type 2 DM occurs predominantly in women.

F. The incidence of type 2 DM is increasing because of the increase in obesity and sedentary lifestyle.

G. There is an increasing prevalence of type 2 DM in developing countries.

H. MODY accounts for 1–5% of cases of DM in the United States.

III. Pathophysiology

A. **Type 2 DM** results from **insulin resistance with a defect in compensatory insulin secretion.**

B. **MODY** results from a **mutation in any of the 6 different genes that are expressed in the β cells of the pancreas.**

C. Nuclear respiratory factor and peroxisome proliferator-activated receptor gamma coactivator-1-dependent oxidative metabolic pathways may play a central and potentially primary role in the pathogenesis of type 2 DM.

IV. Risk Factors

A. **Genetic factor** aggravated by sedentary lifestyle and abdominal visceral obesity

B. **Gestational diabetes** or a mother who delivers an infant larger than 4 kg (9 lb)

C. Persons of African American, Hispanic American, Native American, Asian American, and Pacific Islander descent

D. **Older than 45 years**

E. Previously identified impaired glucose tolerance (IGT) (can increase risk)

F. Hypertension with a blood pressure of ≥ 140/90 mm Hg

G. HDL cholesterol level of ≤ 0.90 mmol/L and/or triglyceride level of ≥ 2.82 mmol/L

H. Polycystic ovary syndrome

V. Clinical Presentation

A. **Symptoms**

1. Polyuria, polydipsia, polyphagia
2. Weight loss
3. Weakness
4. Fatigue
5. Frequent infections
6. Complications (eg, nephropathy, neuropathy, and retinopathy)

B. **Signs**

1. Elevated blood pressure
2. Centripetal obesity
3. Sensory deficit related to peripheral neuropathy
4. Infections (eg, candidal vaginitis)

CLINICAL SKILLS TIP

Consider type 2 DM in the setting of a patient with unexplained fatigue, hypertension, and peripheral neuropathy.

VI. Differential Diagnosis

A. **Type 1 DM**

B. **Other Types of DM**

1. Genetic defects of β-cell function
2. Genetic defects in insulin action
3. Diseases of exocrine pancreas
4. Endocrinopathies
5. Drug or chemical induced
6. Infections
7. Immune-mediated
8. Genetic syndromes sometimes associated with DM

C. **Gestational DM**

RULE OUT

Patients with type 2 DM may have silent cardiac ischemia. When caring for a patient who has type 2 DM, always consider cardiac ischemia even when the patient presents with a history and physical examination not specifically related to the cardiovascular system.

VII. Diagnostic Findings

A. Laboratory Studies

1. **Urinalysis**
   a. Glucosuria
   b. Ketonuria
2. **Blood testing procedures**
   a. **Glucose tolerance test**
      (1) **Methodology and normal fasting glucose:** Plasma and serum from venous blood samples have an advantage over whole blood for providing values for glucose that are independent of hematocrit and that reflect the glucose concentration to which body tissues are exposed.
      (2) **Criteria for laboratory confirmation of DM:** If the fasting plasma glucose level is ≥ 126 mg/dL on 1 or more occasions, further evaluation of the patient using a glucose challenge is unnecessary. If the fasting plasma glucose is < 126 mg/dL in suspected cases, a standardized oral glucose tolerance test (OGTT) may be completed (Table 11–1).
   b. **Serum fructosamine**
   c. **Ongoing management and monitoring studies**
      (1) **Glycated hemoglobin (hemoglobin A_1) measurements:** Glycated hemoglobin is abnormally high in diabetics who have chronic hyperglycemia and reflects their metabolic control. This can be used to monitor a patient's blood glucose level over a 3-month period.
      (2) Self-monitoring of blood glucose
      (3) Continuous glucose monitoring systems
3. **Lipoprotein abnormalities:** In type 2 DM, moderately deficient control of hyperglycemia is associated with an increase in LDL cholesterol and serum triglycerides and little if any decrease in HDL cholesterol.

VIII. Treatment (Figures 11–1, 11–2, and 11–3)

A. Diet and Exercise

1. In **obese patients,** the major goal of diet therapy is **weight reduction** by caloric restriction and exercise.

Table 11–1. Criteria for oral glucose tolerance test (OGTT).

OGTT	Normal Glucose Tolerance	Impaired Glucose Tolerance	Diabetes Mellitus
Fasting plasma glucose	< 110 mg/dL	110–125 mg/dL	≥ 126 mg/dL
Two hours after glucose load	< 140 mg/dL	≥ 140 mg/dL but < 200 mg/dL	≥ 200 mg/dL

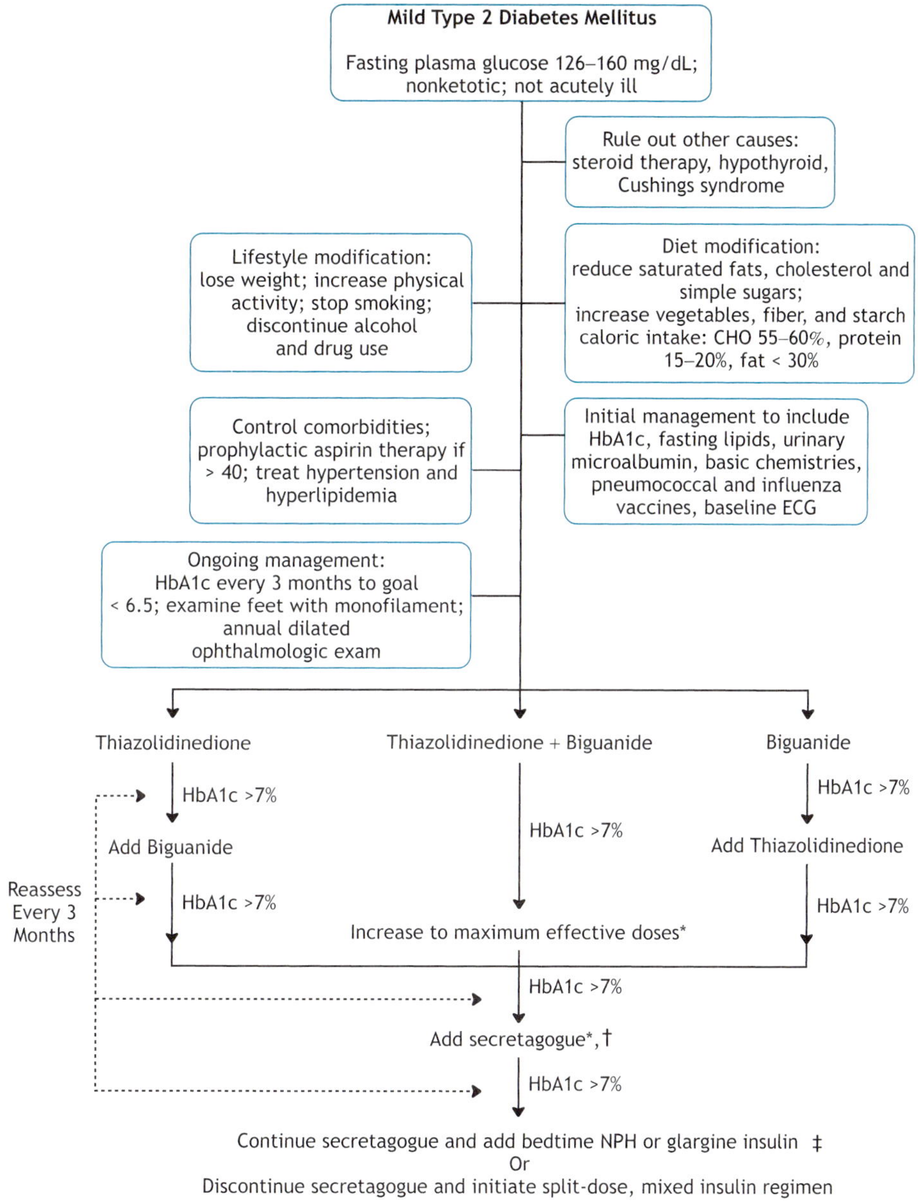

Biguanides are contraindicated in patients with renal disease or dysfunction (as suggested by serum creatinine levels ≥1.5 mg/dL [males], ≥1.4 mg/dL [females), or abnormal creatinine clearance), congestive heart failure requiring pharmacologic treatment, and acute or chronic metabolic acidosis. Thiazolidinediones, alone or in combination with other antidiabetic agents, can cause fluid retention, which may exacerbate or lead to heart failure.

*Sulfonylureas may potentiate or cause hypoglycemia and their use should therefore be reserved, whereas thiazolidinediones and biguanides, alone or in combination with each other, have rarely been shown to cause hypoglycemia.
† If hypoglycemia occurs, back-titrate or discontinue the secretagogue.
‡ Reassess in 3 months, if HbA1c >7%, discontinue secretagogue and initiate split-dose, mixed insulin regimen.

Figure 11–1 Treatment of the patient with mild type 2 diabetes mellitus.

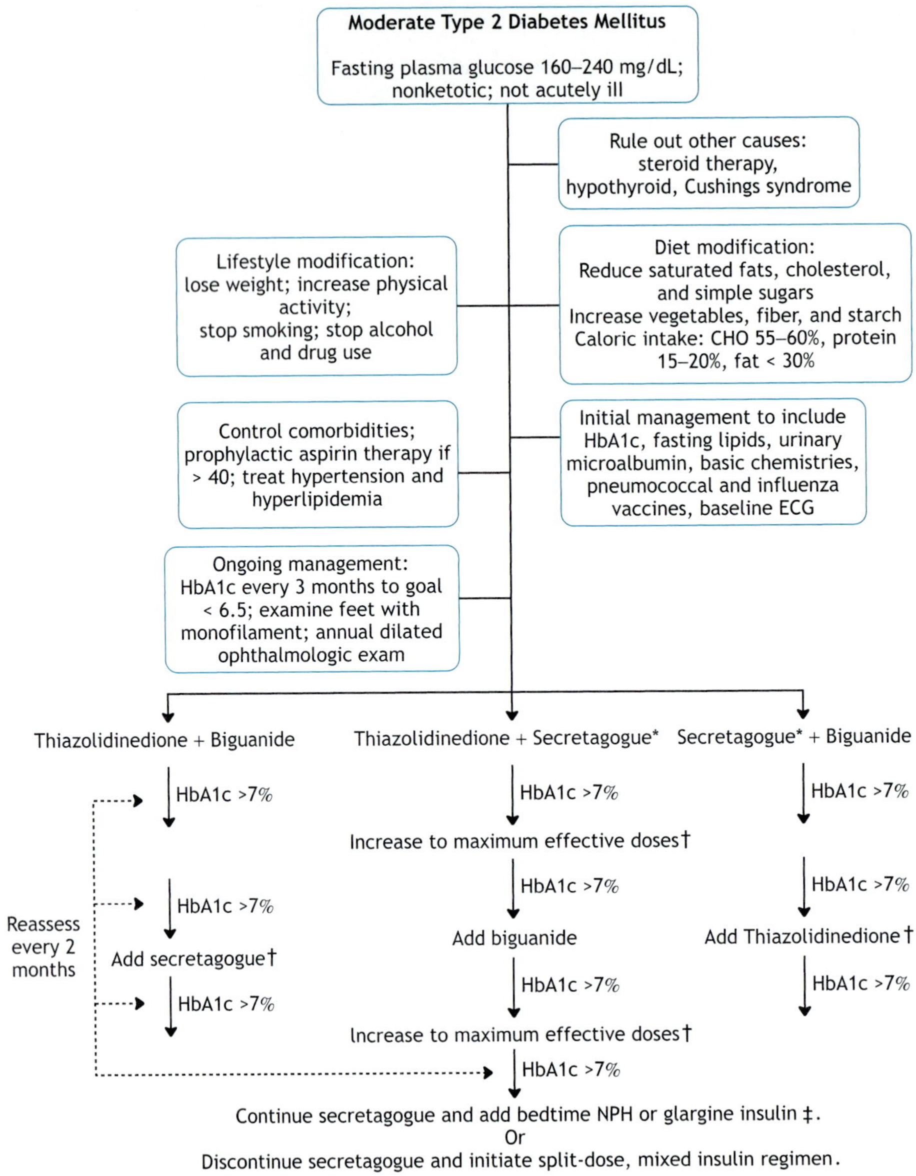

Biguanides are contraindicated in patients with renal disease or dysfunction (as suggested by serum creatinine levels ≥1.5 mg/dL [males], ≥1.4 mg/dL [females], or abnormal creatinine clearance), congestive heart failure requiring pharmacologic treatment, and acute or chronic metabolic acidosis. Thiazolidinediones, alone or in combination with other antidiabetic agents, can cause fluid retention, which may exacerbate or lead to heart failure.

*Sulfonylureas may potentiate or cause hypoglycemia and their use should therefore be reserved, whereas thiazolidinediones and biguanides, alone or in combination with each other, have rarely been shown to cause hypoglycemia.

† If hypoglycemia occurs, back-titrate or discontinue the secretagogue.

‡ Reassess in 3 months, if HbA1c >7%, discontinue secretagogue and initiate split-dose, mixed insulin regimen.

§ If biguanide is contraindicated, add basal insulin, taper off secretagogue, and introduce bolus insulin as needed.

Figure 11–2 Treatment of the patient with moderate type 2 diabetes mellitus.

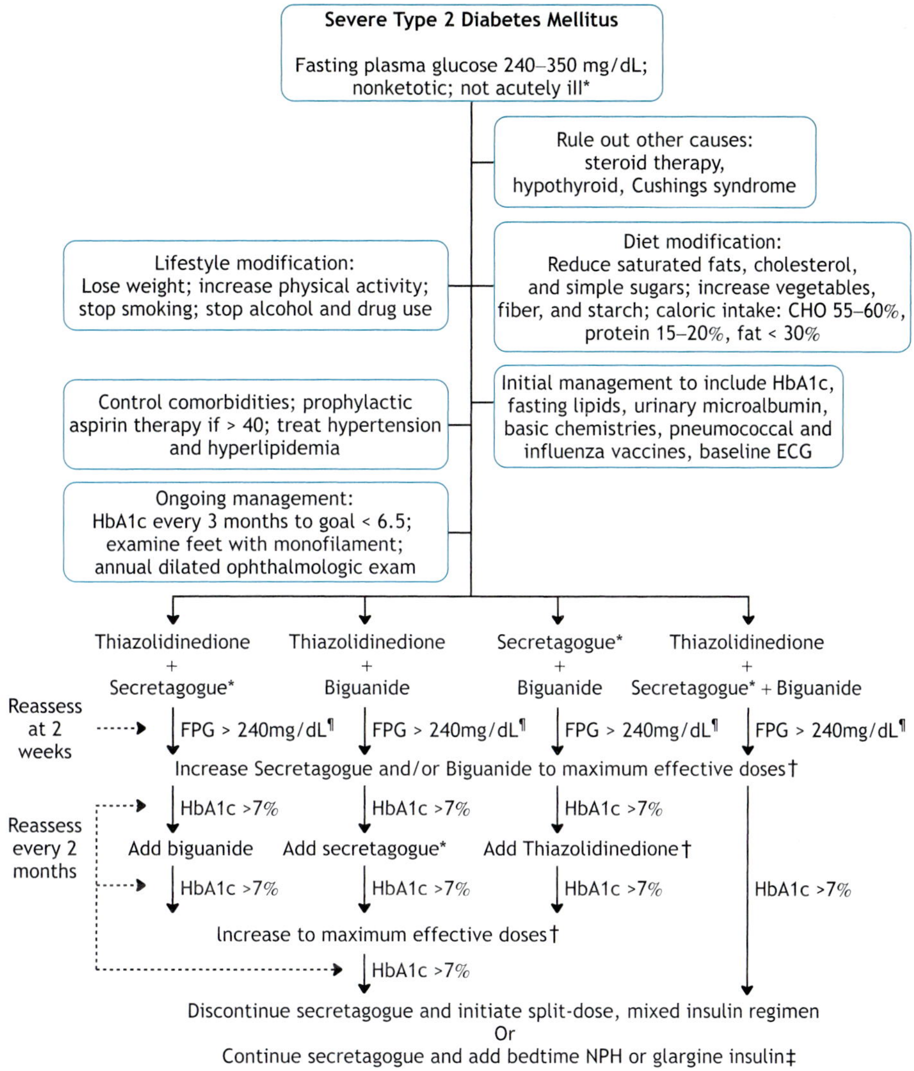

Biguanides are contraindicated in patients with renal disease or dysfunction (as suggested by serum creatinine levels ≥ 1.5 mg/dL [males], ≥ 1.4 mg/dL [females], or abnormal creatinine clearance), congestive heart failure requiring pharmacologic treatment, and acute or chronic metabolic acidosis. Thiazolidinediones, alone or in combination with other antidiabetic agents, can cause fluid retention, which may exacerbate or lead to heart failure.

FPG, fasting plasma glucose; HbA1c, hemoglobinA1c.

*Sulfonylureas may potentiate or cause hypoglycemia and their use should therefore be reserved, whereas thiazolidinediones and biguanides, alone or in combination with each other, have rarely been shown to cause hypoglycemia.

† If hypoglycemia occurs, back-titrate or discontinue the secretagogue.

‡ Reassess in 3 months, if HbA1c >7%, discontinue secretagogue and initiate split-dose, mixed insulin regimen.

§ If biguanide is contraindicated, add basal insulin, taper off secretagogue, and introduce bolus insulin as needed.

If at any lime the patient is symptomatic or acutely ill, consider aggressive, empiric insulin therapy with appropriate guidance.

¶ For patients who remain symptomatic, consider initiating split-dose, mixed insulin regimen and discontinuing secretagogue (if on a secretagogue) or adding bedtime NPH or glargine insulin and continuing secretagogue (if on a secretagogue).

Figure 11–3 Treatment of the patient with severe type 2 diabetes mellitus.

2. Recommend "carbohydrate counting" so the patient can administer 1 unit of regular insulin for each 10–15 g of carbohydrate eaten at a meal.
3. Patients who have type 2 DM should be taught to increase their intake of foods with **noncholesterologenic monounsaturated oils** (eg, olive oil, rapeseed [canola] oil, or nuts and avocados) to limit their carbohydrate intake.
4. Patients should be advised to **limit cholesterol** to 300 mg daily, **protein intake** to 10–20% of total daily calories, and **saturated and polyunsaturated fats** to no more than 8–9% of total caloric intake.
5. Advise patient to eat foods high in **soluble fiber** (eg, oatmeal, cereals, and beans).

B. Drugs that Stimulate Insulin Secretion (Secretagogue)

1. Sulfonylureas (eg, glyburide, glipizide, glimepiride)
2. Meglitinide analogs
3. D-Phenylalanine derivative

C. Drugs that Alter Insulin Action

1. **Biguanide** (metformin) is effective in reducing glycosylated hemoglobin by 1–2% when used as monotherapy or when used in combination with other blood glucose lowering agents or with insulin.
2. **Thiazolidinediones**

D. Drugs that Affect Absorption of Glucose

1. **Acarbose**
   - a. Acarbose is effective in **reducing postprandial hyperglycemia.** It does not stimulate endogenous insulin secretion or promote weight gain.
   - b. Acarbose can be used as a **first-line therapy along with diet and exercise** or in combination with sulfonylureas to lower hemoglobin A1c concentrations.
2. **Miglitol**

E. Drug combinations (eg, glyburide, metformin)

F. Insulin

1. **Ultra-short-acting**
   - a. Insulin aspart
   - b. Insulin lispro
2. **Short-acting**
   - a. Regular Novolin
   - b. Regular Humulin
3. **Intermediate-acting**
   - a. NPH Humulin
   - b. NPH Novolin
4. **Premixed (%NPH/%regular)**
   - a. Novolin 70/30
   - b. Humulin 70/30
   - c. Humalog Mix 75/25 (%NPL/%insulin lispro)
5. **Long-acting**
   - a. Insulin glargine
   - b. Ultralente Humulin

G. Prevention of Complications

1. **Weight loss and exercise**

2. Intensive insulin management
3. Intensive control of blood pressure

IX. Summary Table

Disease	Pathophysiology	Diagnostic Studies	Treatment
Type 2 DM	Insulin resistance	FBS and/or OGTT	Oral hypoglycemic agents, insulin, weight loss
Type I DM	Absolute insulinopenia	FBS or random blood glucose (OGTT rarely necessary)	Insulin
Autoimmune peripheral neuropathy	Autoimmune infiltration of nerve	Nerve conduction velocity	Corticosteroids and other agents

DM, diabetes mellitus; FBS, fasting blood sugar; OGTT, oral glucose tolerance test.

CLINICAL CASE

A 45-year-old woman complains of a burning pain in the entire lower part of her legs and feet that has been present for the past month and is getting worse. It is more sharp then dull, but she mainly says that it burns. It lasts from several minutes to 1 hour and then subsides for many hours. She says that nothing seems to bring it on and nothing makes it go away. She says that there is no weakness. She takes acetaminophen, but it is not effective. Her past history is significant for a recent diagnosis of hypertension and long-standing obesity. She was prescribed 12.5 mg hydrochlorothiazide 1 month ago. She has frequent candidal vaginitis infections. Her family history is significant for hypertension and DM. She does not use alcohol or drugs. Her physical examination is significant for a blood pressure of 138/84 mm Hg and BMI of 29. Heart and lung examinations are normal. Her neurologic examination reveals findings consistent with a peripheral neuropathy of both legs.

Potential etiologies for this patient's peripheral neuropathy include diabetes and alcoholism as well as various autoimmune etiologies. The patient does not use alcohol. Although autoimmune etiologies must be considered, DM is a significantly more common etiology of peripheral neuropathy and should be considered first. Moreover, **the patient's obesity and history of frequent candidal vaginitis are also consistent with a diagnosis of DM.** Had diabetes been considered at the time of the interview or after, we could have asked more questions and we would have asked her about symptoms of polyuria, polydipsia, weight loss, and generalized fatigue. We should also inquire about her pregnancy history to determine if her infants were large-for-gestational age (generally > 4 kg [9 lb]). These additional pieces of her history would help direct us to a diagnosis of DM as the etiology of the peripheral neuropathy.

Before arriving at the diagnosis of peripheral neuropathy, we should examine the thinking involved related to the patient's chief complaint of leg pain. Infectious etiologies are unlikely, particularly in the absence of a history of predisposing trauma and the bilateral nature of the complaint. Although vertebral disk disease could cause the leg pain, the bilateral nature and absence of motor findings make this etiology unlikely. An upper motor neuron lesion could cause the pain, but again the bilateral nature of the pain makes a diagnosis of a single cerebral lesion unlikely. As mentioned above, if the patient were to be diagnosed with something other than DM, the various autoimmune etiologies of a peripheral neuropathy must be investigated.

This patient has type 2 DM. Although peripheral neuropathy is a common complication, generally it is not the presenting complaint. Patients with type 2 DM often have metabolic abnormalities for long periods of time before their symptoms bring them to a physician and a diagnosis is determined. A patient's obesity and insulin resistance often leads to an early increase in insulin secretion by the pancreatic β islet cells. Unfortunately, without weight loss it is generally an inadequate compensatory response, and the patient develops hyperglycemia and the resultant abnormalities. When a patient is pregnant, hyperglycemia crosses the placenta. When the fetus is presented with hyperglycemia, it increases its own secretion of insulin, which leads to macrosomia.

This patient's treatment should include weight loss and oral hypoglycemic agents and/or insulin. It is generally reasonable to offer the patient an opportunity to try weight loss and exercise as the first-line therapy. Even if these do not achieve euglycemia, it is important to praise patients for their behavioral lifestyle changes. If we subsequently add pharmacologic agents to this patient's treatment regimen, she should continue to make lifelong changes and monitor her diet and exercise.

Although there is no single first-line agent, most physicians will start a patient on drugs that stimulate insulin secretion (see VIII B) **or drugs that alter insulin action** (eg, metformin). When initiating pharmacotherapy, it is important for the physician to see a patient who has DM every 3 months and perform a glycohemoglobin test. This test will provide a more accurate understanding of the patient's blood glucose control. If glycohemoglobin remains > 7.0, either increase the current dose of medication (insulin secretagogue or metformin) or add additional agents. **Most patients will need more than one agent to achieve euglycemia. Insulin is often added to the regimen.** When prescribing insulin to patients who have type 2 DM, many physicians will use premixed insulin (eg, 70/30). Although this may be convenient for the patient, it does not allow the physician to "fine-tune" blood glucose control. Many physicians now prescribe a long-acting insulin (eg, insulin glargine), which will help control basal and fasting hyperglycemia. Oral agents can then be combined with the insulin glargine.

Although these medications (insulin secretagogues, metformin, insulin) can correct metabolic abnormalities, DM is a chronic disease. Patients are at risk for multiple long-term sequelae involving the eyes, kidneys, nervous system, and microvascular system, which should be monitored. Stricter control of blood glucose can help delay the onset of these sequelae.

CLINICAL PEARLS

Burning sensation characteristic of peripheral neuropathy, frequent candidal infections, obesity, macrosomia (large- for-gestational age infant), and polyuria and polydipsia would lead the physician to a diagnosis of type 2 DM.

CHAPTER 12
EAR INFECTION

I. Defining Features

A. **Serous Otitis Media**
   1. Pressure in the ear
   2. Hearing loss

B. **Acute and Chronic Otitis Media**
   1. Otalgia
   2. Fever

II. Epidemiology

A. Ear Infections are **most common in children.** By age 7, 93% of children have had at least 1 episode of acute otitis media, and 39% have had 6 or more episodes of acute otitis media.

B. The **peak incidence is between 6 and 18 months of age** and **declines after age 7.**

C. Ear infections are rare in adults.

D. Males are more likely to have acute otitis media than females.

III. Pathophysiology

A. **Serous otitis media** occurs when the auditory tubes remain blocked for a prolonged period; the negative pressure can result in transudation of fluid.

B. **Acute otitis media** is characterized as a **bacterial infection** of the mucosally lined air-containing spaces of the temporal bone. Purulent material forms within the middle ear cleft. This material also forms when the mastoid air cells and petrous apex are pneumatized.

C. **Chronic otitis media** generally occurs as a result of recurrent acute otitis media, although it can follow other diseases and trauma. Generally, there is a perforation of the tympanic membrane. There can also be mucosal changes (eg, polypoid degeneration and granulation tissue) and osseous changes (eg, osteitis and sclerosis).

D. **Serous otitis media** usually occurs in adults following an upper respiratory tract infection or barotrauma.

IV. Risk Factors

A. Bottle feeding while supine

B. Attending day care

C. Formula feeding
D. Smoking in household
E. Male gender
F. Family history of middle ear disease
G. History of otitis media in sibling

V. Clinical Presentation

A. Symptoms and Signs of Acute Otitis Media

1. Earache
2. Runny nose and low grade fever (accompany upper respiratory tract infections)
3. Decreased hearing
4. Otorrhea, if eardrum perforated
5. Unusual irritability
6. Difficulty sleeping
7. Tugging at the ear
8. Loss of balance
9. Fever, although usually afebrile
10. Eardrum mobility decreased (observed by pneumatic otoscopy)
11. Bulging eardrum (observed with otoscopy); opaque, often yellowish fluid; inflammation (redness alone not a reliable sign)

B. Symptoms and Signs of Otitis Media in Infants

1. May be asymptomatic in the first few months of life
2. Irritability, may be only indication of earache
3. Bulging eardrum
4. Opaque, often yellowish fluid; inflamed (redness alone not a reliable sign)

CLINICAL SKILLS TIP

Symptoms of ear infections in infants will be nonspecific. In a child who has fever or non-focal symptoms, the tympanic membrane should be examined. Redness alone is not a reliable sign; look for a bulging or opaque ear drum.

VI. Differential Diagnosis

A. Tympanosclerosis
B. Redness (due to crying)
C. Referred pain from the jaw or teeth (earache with a normal ear examination)

RULE OUT

If acute otitis media is diagnosed in an infant, the physician must be certain that there are no other more serious bacterial infections. Clinical assessment of toxicity is important.

VII. Diagnostic Findings

A. **Laboratory studies:** White blood cell count is higher in bacterial acute otitis media than in sterile acute otitis media.

B. Diagnostic Studies

1. **Tympanometry, acoustic reflexometry, or acoustic reflectometry** can be used to document the presence of fluid in the middle ear.

2. **Tympanocentesis** is recommended for culture of middle ear fluid when other treatments fail. This may be followed by myringotomy.

VIII. Treatment (Figure 12–1; Tables 12–1 and 12–2)

A. Treat **serous otitis media with a short course of an oral corticosteroid** (eg, prednisone 40 mg/d for 7 days). **Oral antibiotics** can also be used, or a **combination of an antibiotic and prednisone** (oral corticosteroid).

B. Treat **acute otitis media with a specific antibiotic** (eg, amoxicillin or erythromycin plus sulfonamide) often **in combination with a nasal decongestant.**

C. For **chronic otitis media, remove infected debris regularly;** use **earplugs** to protect against exposure to water; and apply **topical antibiotic drops** for exacerbations.

D. In most cases, **definitive management of chronic otitis media is surgical** (tympanostomy with pressure equalization tube placement).

E. **Prevention**

1. **Breast-feeding** can decrease the incidence of acute otitis media.
2. **Eliminating cigarette smoke** in the household.
3. Administer the **heptavalent pneumococcal conjugate vaccine** (PCV-78) [with nontoxic diphtheria-toxin analogue carrier protein, CRM197] to help prevent acute otitis media caused by susceptible serotypes.

IX. Summary Table

Condition	Pathophysiology	Diagnostic Studies	Treatment
Acute otitis media	Infectious (viral or bacterial)	Physical examination	Antibiotics
Meningitis	Infectious	Lumbar puncture, CBC, cultures	Antibiotics
Red tympanic membrane due to crying	Vascular filling	Physical examination	None
Serous otitis media	Obstruction	Physical examination; tympanometry	Possibly antibiotics and/or corticosteroids

CLINICAL CASE

A mother brings her 12-month-old infant to the office because he has a low-grade fever and is irritable and has not been eating solid foods for the past 2 days. The boy has been pulling at his left ear. He is breast-feeding without any problems, and his diapers are wet. His sleep has not been interrupted, but he has been crying more than usual during the day. The infant

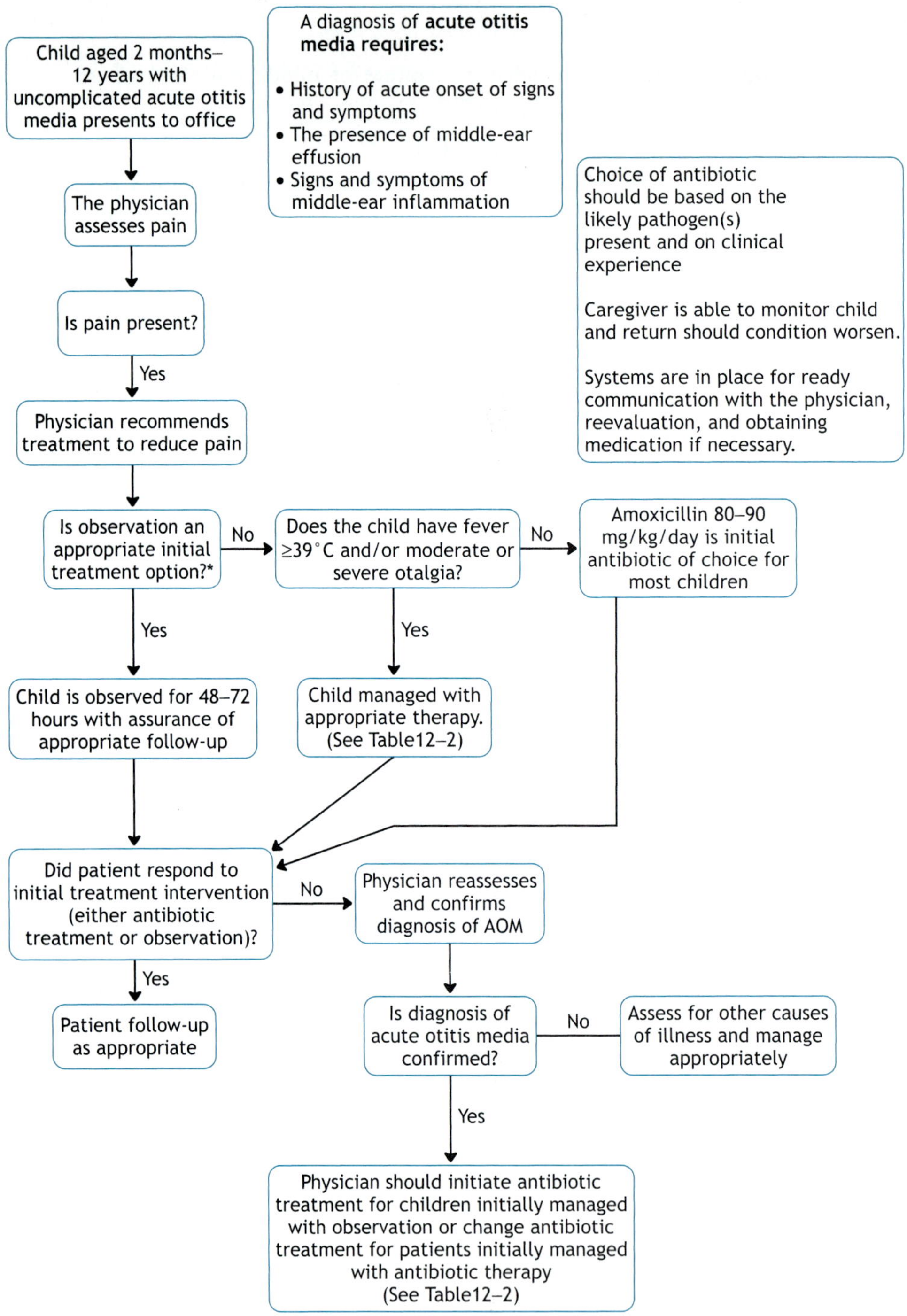

Figure 12–1 Management of the patient with acute otitis media.

Table 12–1. Factors to consider in the treatment of acute otitis media.

• Temperature > 38.6 °C (101.5 °F) within the past 48 hours
• Symptoms suggestive of acute otitis media > 48 hours
• Toxic appearance
• Tympanic membrane of the infected ear not intact
• Recurrent episode of acute otitis media within past 3 months
• Signs of impending perforation in the infected ear, as judged by examining physician
• Coexisting bacterial infection
• Concerns of physician that the family would be unable to seek medical care if the child's clinical status were to worsen
• Concerns of caregiver or physician that the caregiver could not gain an acceptable understanding of the therapeutic plan

is in a day-care program 4 mornings a week. His past history reveals that he weighed 3.4 kg (7 lb 8 oz) at birth. The mother's pregnancy and the vaginal delivery were uncomplicated. The infant has reached all developmental milestones at the appropriate times. He has not been sick and takes no medicines. He has not received his third set of vaccinations and has not been given any of the pneumococcal conjugate vaccines. He is an only child. On physical examination, his temperature is 37.9 °C (100.3 °F), and the remainder of his vital signs are normal. He is sitting quietly in his mother's lap and does not appear toxic. His heart and lung examinations are normal. Otoscopy shows a bulging and opaque left ear drum. His right ear is normal. There is a yellowish discharge from his nose. Although he is somewhat irritable during the ear examination, he was easily consoled by his mother. A brief neurologic examination indicates that he is alert and interactive with his mother. He moves all extremities. The mother says that he has just begun walking.

As with many infants, this infant presents with essentially nonspecific complaints other than the apparent otalgia. A thorough physical examination is essential and an important component is the impression of the examiner. **This child presents with many of the signs and symptoms related to acute otitis media** (see V). Equally important is the lack of findings consistent with a more worrisome diagnosis such as bacterial meningitis or pneumonia. Ultimately, the low-grade fever, the likely exposure to a viral illness at day care, and the physical findings in the ear assure the diagnosis of acute otitis media.

When thinking about this infant and a differential diagnosis, almost all possible etiologies will be infection-related. Congenital etiologies are always of concern in infants; however, the relatively acute onset accompanied by fever would make these etiologies less likely. **Causes that are metabolic- or endocrine-related must also be considered in a presentation of non-focal complaints.** However, the otalgia directs the physician to the ear as the first line of thinking. Regarding infectious etiologies, the first task for the physi-

TABLE 12–2. Recommended antibacterial agents for patients who are being treated initially with antibacterial agents or have failed 48–72 hours of observation or initial management with antibacterial agents.

Temperature ≥ 39 °C (102.2 °F) and/or Severe Otalgia	At Diagnosis for Patients being Treated Initially With Antibacterial Agents		Clinically Defined Treatment Failure at 48–72 Hours After Initial Management With Observation Option		Clinically Defined Treatment Failure at 48–72 Hours After Initial Management With Antibacterial Agents	
	Recommended	Alternative for Penicillin Allergy	Recommended	Alternative for Penicillin Allergy	Recommended	Alternative for Penicillin Allergy
No	Amoxicillin, 80–90 mg/kg/day	Non-type I: cefdinir, cefuroxime, cefpodoxime; type I: azithromycin, clarithromycin	Amoxicillin, 80–90 mg/kg/day	Non-type I: cefdinir, cefuroxime, cefpodoxime; type I: azithromycin, clarithromycin	Amoxicillin/ clavulanate, 90 mg/kg/day amoxicillin component, with 6.4 mg/kg/day clavulanate	Non-type I: ceftriaxone, 3 days; type I: clindamycin
Yes	Amoxicillin/ clavulanate, 90 mg/kg/day amoxicillin, with 6.4 mg/kg/day clavulanate	Ceftriaxone, 1 or 3 days	Amoxicillin/ clavulanate, 90 mg/kg/day amoxicillin, with 6.4 mg/kg/day clavulanate	Ceftriaxone, 1 or 3 days	Ceftriaxone, 3 days	Tympanocentesis, clindamycin

cian is to triage between a seriously ill infant and the one who is not seriously ill. Again, look at vital signs and indicators of the clinical impression of toxicity. Having triaged this infant, **the physician then should consider whether the cause is viral, bacterial, or fungal.** Although the physician did not perform a culture of the ear effusion, the **decision to consider it bacterial is based on the appearance of the tympanic membrane,** but this cannot be considered certain, and there is no diagnostic test or procedure (other than tympanocentesis and culture) to ensure that it is bacterial. Spontaneous resolution rates are between 78–80% within 7–14 days.

This patient has acute otitis media. The likely etiology relates to the infant's exposure to a virus of the upper respiratory tract at day care. This viral infection then becomes superinfected with bacteria. Although pneumococcal conjugate vaccine does not prevent all acute otitis media, its absence in this infant was definitely a risk factor. Smoking in the household (which we should have inquired about from the mother) would also increase this child's risk of acute otitis media. The next clinical challenges arise if the child develops chronic otitis media or serous otitis media. These infections can result in serious problems, such as hearing loss and difficulties in school.

At future visits, **the physician should differentiate between recurrent otitis and resistant otitis.** Prevention can include the elimination of smoking in the household, switching from bottle-feeding to breast-feeding, giving pneumococcal conjugate vaccine, and prescribing suppressive doses of antibiotics.

CLINICAL PEARLS

It is critical to avoid inappropriate use of antibiotics.

CHAPTER 13
HEADACHE

I. Defining Features

A. Headaches are divided into two categories: primary headaches and secondary headaches.
   1. **Primary headaches** have **no causal disease** and include migraine, tension, and cluster.
   2. **Secondary headaches** are due to a **causal disease** such as a brain tumor, meningitis, or subarachnoid hemorrhage.

B. The intensity, quality, and site of pain are factors that can help define the underlying cause.

C. **Migraine headaches** have premonitory symptoms, visual sensory symptoms or motor symptoms, unilateral throbbing pain, and nausea and vomiting.

D. The pain in **tension headaches** is holocephalic and can be related to stress.

E. **Cluster headaches** are characterized by episodes of recurrent, nocturnal, unilateral, retro-orbital searing pain.
   1. Attacks may occur at the same time on consecutive days (cluster).
   2. An attack frequently occurs within 90 minutes of falling asleep (corresponding to the first REM-stage sleep).

F. Patients with **secondary headaches** invariably have focal neurologic deficits or accompanying symptoms such as nausea or vomiting.

II. Epidemiology

A. Migraine Headache
   1. About **18% of adult females** and **6% of adult males have migraines.**
   2. The **predominant age of onset of migraines is childhood;** incidence increases in early adolescence and continues to increase up to age 40, and then decreases with age.
   3. **Prevalence of migraines is highest in adult women,** individuals aged 25–55 years, and individuals from low income households.

B. Tension Headache
   1. Tension headaches are very **common.**
   2. About **60% of persons who have tension headaches begin to have them after age 20,** but it is unusual to begin after age 50.

C. **Cluster Headache**

1. **About 0.2% of the population has cluster headaches.**
2. Cluster headaches are **more common in men** than in woman, with a ratio of 6:1.
3. The mean age for cluster headaches in men is **age 30,** and occurs later in women.

III. Pathophysiology

A. **Migraine headache:** The causes of migraines are unknown but may be due to

1. **Neuronal disease** with vascular disruption as an epiphenomenon of underlying neurochemical disruption
2. **Serotonin, dopamine, glutamate and norepinephrine metabolic abnormalities**
3. **Neurogenic inflammation** and regional disruption of cerebral and/or extracranial blood flow

B. **Tension headache:** The causes of tension headaches are unknown but may be due to

1. Tension headaches are thought to be initiated by a peripheral mechanism, most likely **increased input from the myofascial nociceptors.**
2. Chronic tension headaches may be caused by an **impaired supraspinal modulation of the incoming stimuli.**

C. **Cluster headache:** The exact causes of cluster headaches are unknown but may be due to

1. Disruption of the circadian rhythm based on the hypothalamus
2. Disturbed autoregulation of cerebral arteries
3. Disorder of serotonin metabolism or transmission in the central nervous system (CNS)
4. Disorder of histamine concentrations or receptors

IV. Risk Factors

A. **Migraine Headache**

1. **Specific foods** such as red wine, cured or processed meats, or aged cheese; alcohol; not eating regular meals; hormonal changes; or excessive sleep, fatigue, emotional stress, and emotional let down (relief of stress)
2. **Medications,** such as estrogen replacement therapy, oral contraceptive pills, or vasodilators
3. **Family history of migraine**
4. **Female gender**
5. **Young age**
6. History of childhood cyclic vomiting, cyclic abdominal pain, motion sickness

B. **Tension Headache**

1. **Excess caffeine**
2. **Obstructive sleep apnea**
3. **Rebound headaches:** medications such as barbiturates, sedatives, or narcotics

C. **Cluster Headache**

1. **Male** gender
2. **Older than age 30 years**

3. **Small amounts of vasodilators** such as alcohol (< 4 oz) or nitroglycerin
4. **Previous history of head trauma or surgery**
5. If a **first-degree relative has cluster headaches,** a person is 2–18 times more likely to have cluster headaches.

V. Clinical Presentation

A. Symptoms of migraine headaches may vary from patient to patient or from attack to attack. The 5 phases of a migraine are

1. **Premonitory symptoms** (experienced by 50–80% of patients)
   a. Various "warning signs" that precede migraines are frequently characterized by mood disruptions (eg, euphoria, irritability, and depression), fatigue, muscle tension, food cravings, bloating, yawning, or subtle disruption of sensory processing.
   b. These symptoms often are not recognized by patients as being associated with migraine headache.
2. **Aura**
   a. **Visual disruptions** are most common and include scotoma, hemianopsia, geometric visual patterns, and occasionally hallucinations.
   b. **Somatosensory disruption** in the face or upper extremities is common.
   c. **Headache typically begins within 1 hour of aura resolution.**
3. **Headache**
   a. A **headache usually begins with mild pain** that escalates to a **unilateral throbbing pain** that lasts anywhere from 4 to 72 hours.
   b. It is **intensified by movement.**
   c. Symptoms are associated with **systemic manifestations** (eg, nausea, vomiting, diarrhea, photophobia, phonophobia, muscle tenderness, lightheadedness, and vertigo).
4. **Headache Termination**
   a. If untreated, usually **termination of pain occurs with sleep.**
   b. Occasionally, vomiting or strong emotional experiences abort the headache.
5. **Postdrome**
   a. **Headache pain is resolved.**
   b. Other manifestations may linger, including food intolerance, impaired concentration, fatigue, or muscle soreness.

B. Symptoms of Tension Headaches

1. Bilateral headache (90% of patients)
2. Fronto-occipital or generalized pain
3. Dull, pressing, or band-like pain
4. Intensity varies throughout the day
5. Often present upon arising or shortly thereafter
6. Chronic tension headache duration > 5 years (75% of patients)
7. Insomnia
8. Teeth grinding
9. Difficulty concentrating
10. Muscular tightness or stiffness in neck and occipital and frontal regions

C. Symptoms and Signs of Cluster Headaches

1. **Sudden onset of severe headache**

2. Headache reaches crescendo within 15 minutes, lasts < 3 hours
3. Unilateral, oculotemporal, or oculofrontal pain; rarely in other locations
4. Severe, piercing, boring, exploding, penetrating, occasionally throbbing pain
5. Ipsilateral partial Horner syndrome (ptosis and miosis)
6. Lacrimation, injected conjunctiva, rhinorrhea
7. Bradycardia
8. Nausea, perspiration, restlessness and agitation during attacks

CLINICAL SKILLS TIPS

Warning symptoms and signs of headache associated with significant underlying disease:

- *Sudden onset, no previous history of this type of headache, change in mental status, concomitant facial infection, and headache related to vigorous exercise.*
- *Fever (meningitis or encephalitis); reduced level of consciousness, nuchal rigidity, preretinal hemorrhages (subarachnoid hemorrhage); papilledema, focal neurologic signs, varying level of consciousness (intracranial mass); tenderness over pulseless, nodular, tender temporal artery (temporal arteritis); ataxia, altered mental status, loss of consciousness (acute hydrocephalus); focal neurologic findings, impaired mental status, cranial nerve dysfunction (cerebral vascular attack, known as CVA).*

VI. Differential Diagnosis (Figure 13–1)

A. Migraine Headache

1. Other primary headache disorders
2. Secondary headaches, including tumor, infection, vascular pathology, or prescription or illicit drug use (eg, cocaine)
3. Drug-seeking patients
4. Psychiatric disease
5. Migraine symptoms similar to certain types of epilepsy (rarely)

B. Tension Headache

1. Cervical spondylosis
2. Temporomandibular joint (TMJ) syndrome
3. Caffeine dependency
4. Nonprescription analgesic dependency
5. Depression
6. Head injury
7. Severe anemia or polycythemia
8. Dental disease
9. Chronic sinusitis
10. Refractive error
11. Hypoxia
12. Temporal arteritis
13. Migraine

C. Cluster Headache

1. Other head and neck pathology
2. Migraine
3. Trigeminal and other facial neuralgias
4. Chronic paroxysmal hemicrania (probably a cluster variant)
5. Temporal arteritis
6. Pheochromocytoma

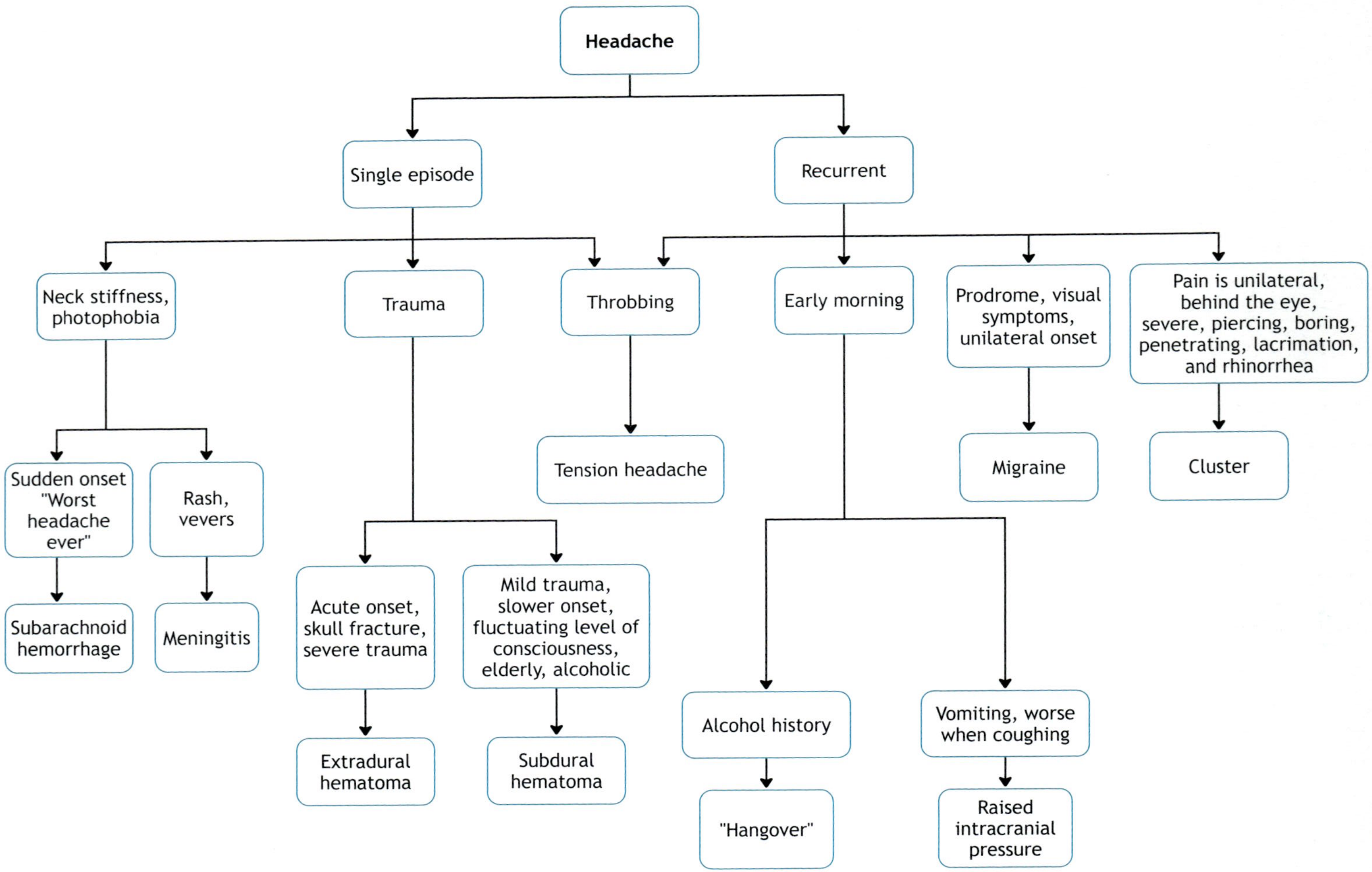

Figure 13-1. Differential diagnosis of headache.

RULE OUT

Secondary causes of headache must be ruled out when suggested by signs and symptoms (see V and VI). Consider meningitis, intracranial bleed, temporal arteritis, stroke, or tumor.

VII. Diagnostic Findings

A. Laboratory Studies

1. **Tension Headache**
   a. Complete blood cell count (CBC)
   b. Blood chemistries
   c. Thyroid studies
   d. Erythrocyte sedimentation rate (ESR) in anyone older than age 50

B. Imaging Studies

1. **Migraine Headache**
   a. **Head CT or MRI** may be indicated for a patient older than age 50 who has **new onset of headache.**
   b. **Head CT scan or MRI** may be necessary for a patient who has a **change in an established headache pattern.**
2. **Tension Headache**
   a. **X-rays of cervical spine** can be helpful to determine if osteoarthritis is causing the headache.
   b. **Head CT scan or MRI** may be necessary only **when headache pattern has recently changed** or there is a **positive finding on a neurologic examination.**

VIII. Treatment

A. Migraine Headache

1. A combined therapy of avoidance of any precipitating factors and prophylactic or symptomatic pharmacologic treatment (if necessary) is used in the management of migraines.
2. **Symptomatic Therapy**
   a. During acute attacks, it may be helpful for the patient to **rest in a dark, quiet room** until the pain subsides. A simple analgesic such as acetaminophen taken immediately often provides relief.
   b. **Cafergot,** a combination of ergotamine tartrate (1 mg) and caffeine (100 mg), is sometimes helpful.
   c. **Triptans** (selective serotonin-$_1$ receptor agonist), including sumatriptan and zolmitriptan, are mainstays of treatment. **Sumatriptan should be avoided during pregnancy.**
3. **Prophylactic therapy** can be used to prevent recurrent migraines.
   a. Aspirin
   b. Propranolol
   c. Amitriptyline or imipramine
   d. Sertraline or fluoxetine
   e. Ergonovine maleate
   f. Cyproheptadine
   g. Clonidine
   h. Verapamil

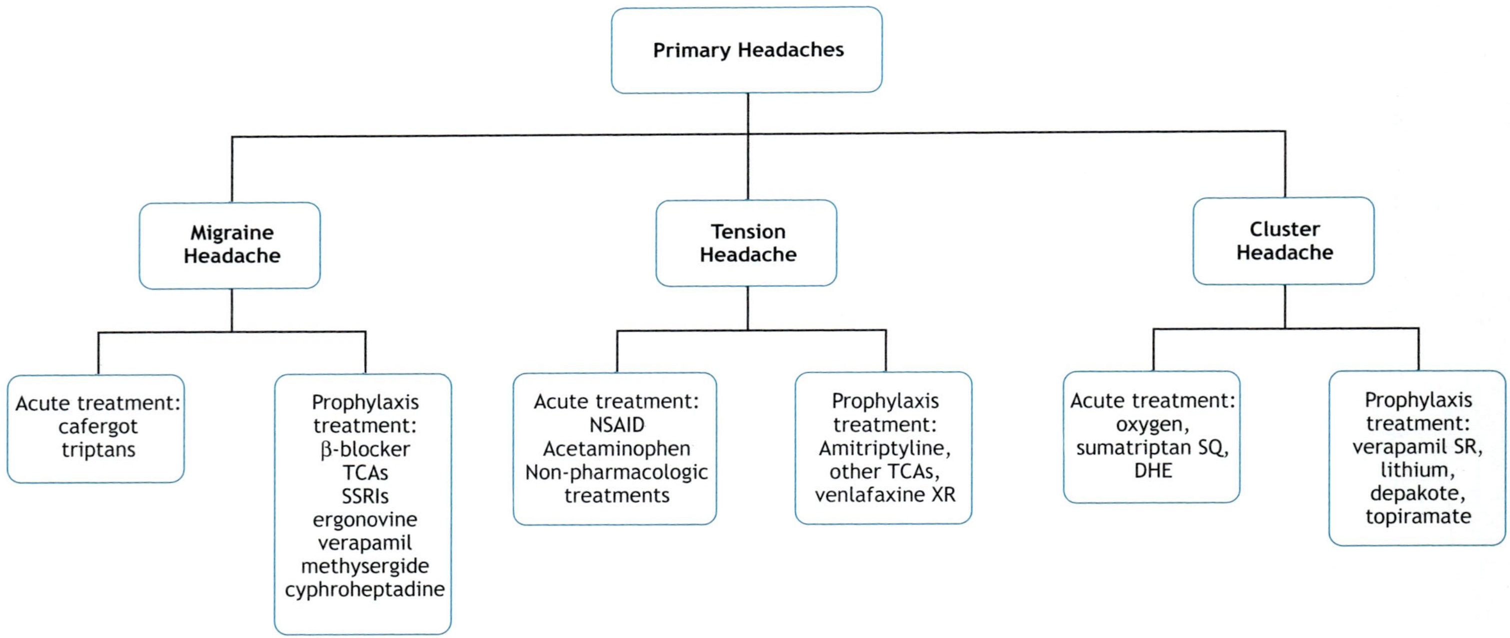

Figure 13-2. Treatment for primary headaches.

B. Tension Headaches

1. **Relief from pain may be obtained through induced relaxation:** massage, hot baths, and biofeedback.
2. **Pharmacotherapy**
   a. **Acute attack: Nonsteroidal anti-inflammatory drugs (NSAIDs)**
      (1) Naproxen sodium (Naprosyn, Aleve) 500 mg/bid
      (2) Fenoprofen calcium (Nalfon) 600 mg/day (200 mg q 4–6 h)
      (3) Ibuprofen (Motrin, Advil) 400 mg/tid
      (4) Ketoprofen (Orudis) 50 mg/tid
   b. **Chronic tension headache**: **Prophylaxis antidepressants**
      (1) Amitriptyline (Elavil) 50–100 mg/day
      (2) Desipramine (Norpramin) 50–100 mg/day
      (3) Imipramine (Tofranil) 50–100 mg/day
      (4) Nortriptyline (Pamelor) 25–50 mg/day

C. Cluster Headache

1. **Alcohol, bright and glaring lights, excessive emotion, and stress** can precipitate attacks and should be avoided during cluster periods.
2. **Avoid narcotic analgesics,** especially oral preparations.
3. **Avoid tobacco** (high predilection for tobacco abuse in this population); tobacco can make patients more refractory to therapy.
4. **Medications**
   a. **Acute**
      (1) Subcutaneous sumatriptan
      (2) Dihydroergotamine
      (3) Ergotamine tartrate aerosol
      (4) Butorphanol tartrate (as nasal spray)
      (5) Ergotamine tartrate (can give as rectal suppository)
      (6) 100% O_2 (7 L/min for 15 min)
   b. **Prophylaxis**
      (1) Propranolol
      (2) Amitriptyline
      (3) Valproate
      (4) Cyproheptadine
      (5) Lithium carbonate (monitor plasma levels)
      (6) Verapamil
      (7) Methysergide

IX. Summary Table

Condition	Pathophysiology	Diagnostic Studies	Treatment
Migraine headache	Vascular	Physical examination; if indicated, head CT scan ESR, x-ray of cervical spine	Triptans, ergotamines, acetaminophen

(*continued*)

IX. Summary Table (continued)

Condition	Pathophysiology	Diagnostic Studies	Treatment
Tension headache	Initiated by a peripheral mechanism, most likely increased input from the myofascial nociceptors Chronic tension headaches may be an impaired supraspinal modulation of the incoming stimuli	Physical examination; if indicated, head CT scan, ESR, x-ray of cervical spine	NSAIDs
Cluster headache	Unknown/vascular	Physical examination; if indicated head CT scan, ESR, x-ray of cervical spine	Triptans, ergots, O_2, nasal butorphanol, dihydro-ergotamine
Secondary headache (multiple etiologies)	Varied	CBC, LP, CT scan of head, cultures of spinal fluid and blood	As indicated

CBC, complete blood cell count; CT, computer tomography; ESR, erythrocyte sedimentation rate; LP, lumbar puncture.

CLINICAL CASE

A 27-year-old woman presents with a headache that she describes as "horrible." She says that she was in her usual state of good health until last evening when the headache began, which she describes as band-like around her head into the back of her neck. Although occasionally the pain feels like it throbs, it is mainly a tight and squeezing pain. She states that she has had headaches in the past, but this is much worse. She would rate it as a 7 on a scale of 1–10. She has taken acetaminophen, which has helped a little, but she still has pain. She felt somewhat better lying down, but the headache was still present when she awoke this morning. She denies any focal weakness or sensory loss; she has no rhinorrhea or HEENT symptoms. Although she would prefer to be in a dark room, the light does not hurt her eyes. When asked about her daily life, she says that she is a single mother on welfare and that life has been extremely stressful recently, with yesterday being particularly bad. She has no significant past medical history. Her mother and both of her sisters get headaches. On physical examination, she appears in pain and is holding her head in her hands. Her vital signs are normal. Her fundoscopic examination is normal, and there are no signs of papilledema. Her neck is supple, but it hurts when she moves her head. Heart, lung, and neurologic examinations are normal.

The first task in evaluating this patient is for the physician to determine if the patient has a primary or a secondary headache. Primary headaches include tension, migraine, and cluster headaches. The possible etiologies for secondary headaches are extensive, including meningitis, cerebral neoplasm or aneurysm, and subarachnoid hemorrhage. Many of the signs and symptoms of a secondary headache are extremely serious, and the physician must determine early in the examination if the patient has a secondary headache.

Warnings signs of a secondary headache include the signs listed in the *Clinical Skills Tips.* Those signs and symptoms would help to direct the physician to the following **diagnosis:**

1. **Subacute and/or progressive headaches,** which worsen over time (months) may represent a progressive intracranial lesion such as a tumor, subdural hematoma, or hydrocephalus.
2. A **new or different type of headache** may represent subarachnoid hemorrhage, meningitis, or hypertensive encephalopathy.
3. **Any headache of maximum severity at onset** may represent subarachnoid hemorrhage.
4. **Headache of new onset in a person older than age 50** may represent giant cell arteritis or other systemic disorders.
5. Evidence such as **fever, hypertension myalgias, weight loss, or scalp tenderness** may represent a systemic disorder.
6. Presence of **neurologic signs** that may suggest a secondary cause may represent an intracranial lesion.
7. **Seizures** may represent a space occupying lesion, infection, stroke, or metabolic derangement.

The absence of focal neurologic deficits, fever, papilledema, and meningismus in this patient make it seem significantly unlikely that she has a secondary headache. Our task then is to differentiate among the three primary headaches. We need to take a detailed history and perform a physical examination.

The **history** should include the following elements:

1. **Temporal profile:** What is the time from onset to peak; usual time of onset (season, month, menstrual cycle, week, hour of day); frequency and duration? Is it stable or changing over the past 6 months?
2. **Autonomic features:** Is there nasal stuffiness, rhinorrhea, tearing, eyelid ptosis, or edema?
3. **Descriptive characteristics:** Is it pulsatile, throbbing, pressing, or sharp?
4. **Location:** Is it unilateral or bilateral? Does it change sides?
5. **Severity:** How bad is it on a scale of 1–10?
6. **Precipitating features:** What brings it on?
7. **Aggravating and alleviating factors:** What makes it better? What makes it worse?
8. **Pharmacologic and non-pharmacologic treatments:** Are there any medications that are effective or ineffective?
9. **History of other medical problems:** Are there any ongoing medical problems?
10. **Aura:** Is there an aura that precedes the headache?

The **physical examination** should include the following:

1. **Vital signs:** blood pressure, pulse, respirations, and temperature
2. **Evaluation of the extracranial structure** such as carotid arteries, sinuses, scalp arteries, and cervical paraspinal muscles

3. **Examination of the neck in flexion** versus lateral rotation for meningeal irritation.
4. **Focused neurologic examination** should include
   - **Assessment of patient's awareness and consciousness,** presence of confusion, and memory impairment
   - **Ophthalmologic examination** to include pupillary symmetry and reactivity, optic fundi, visual fields, and ocular motility
   - **Cranial nerve examination** to include corneal reflexes, facial sensation, and facial symmetry
   - **Symmetric muscle tone, strength, or deep tendon reflexes**
   - **Sensation**
   - **Plantar responses**
   - **Gait, arm, and leg coordination**

Evaluating the signs and symptoms of our patient would assist in formulating a **differential diagnosis.** Cluster headaches more commonly occur in men and are associated with a severe, piercing pain, lacrimation, injected conjunctiva, nasal stuffiness, and rhinorrhea. Patients who have migraine headaches often have premonitory symptoms, an aura, and a headache that is more commonly throbbing and unilateral. There is often associated nausea, vomiting, and photophobia. Although our patient experienced some of these symptoms, her headache is less likely a migraine and more likely a tension headache. Tension headaches are more commonly bilateral, fronto-occipital, and band-like, as she describes. There is associated muscular tightness or stiffness in the neck. Intensity can vary throughout the day, and it is often present on arising, as she has described. Although patients are not always able to identify stressors, these headaches are associated with stressful life events. Our patient seems to have a stressful life and states that the last day has been even more stressful.

This patient's **treatment** includes both the acute component as well as the possibility of prophylaxis, because tension headaches often become chronic. Acutely, some patients find biofeedback or other methods of induced relaxation helpful. Medications generally include NSAIDs. Prophylaxis for chronic tension headaches generally includes anti-depressants (see VIII B). Over a period of time, many patients can learn to identify stressors that initiate headaches and can work to avoid these situations or at least begin acute treatment early.

CLINICAL PEARLS

Bilateral, fronto-occipital, and band-like character of the headache in the absence of focal neurologic deficits and a patient with stressful life events helps the physician diagnose tension headache.

CHAPTER 14

HEALTH PROMOTION, DISEASE PREVENTION, AND ADULT WELL CARE

I. Introduction: This chapter does not address a symptom or disease. It focuses on one of the most important things we do as family physicians: health promotion and disease prevention. At times, patients visit us for an annual "check-up." However, we must often integrate these critically important activities into the regular "sick" visit. This chapter presents a model to help us as physicians perform this important work. Many tables are included that summarize information on etiology and adult well care.

II. Epidemiology

A. Physicians are providing preventive services in only one third of acute care visits.

B. **Only one half of the population in the United States is currently receiving key preventive care services** such as tobacco cessation counseling, vision screening, regular screening for colorectal cancer, and counseling about vaccinations.

C. A recent study of 4000 patients indicates that only 55% of screening procedures, 24% of immunizations, and 9% of health-habit counseling milestones were up-to-date.

III. Procedures: The mnemonic **RISE** can be used as a guide to providing preventive health care services to adults: ***R***isk identification, ***I***mmunizations, ***S***creening, and ***E***ducation (Figure 14–1).

CLINICAL SKILLS TIP

*Use the RISE mnemonic when providing preventive health care services to adults: **R**isk identification, **I**mmunizations, **S**creening, and **E**ducation.*

A. **Risk identification** can be addressed through regularly published data that indicate the leading causes of death by age and gender. These data can help the physician to tailor the prevention and educational activities for the individual patient (Tables 14–1 through Table 14–7).

B. **Immunizations** reduce disease incidence. Table 14–8 summarizes recommended immunizations for adults. (See Chapter 23 for recommended immunizations for infants, children, and adolescents.)

C. **Screening for asymptomatic disease:** The 5 criteria used to justify the use of preventive screening are

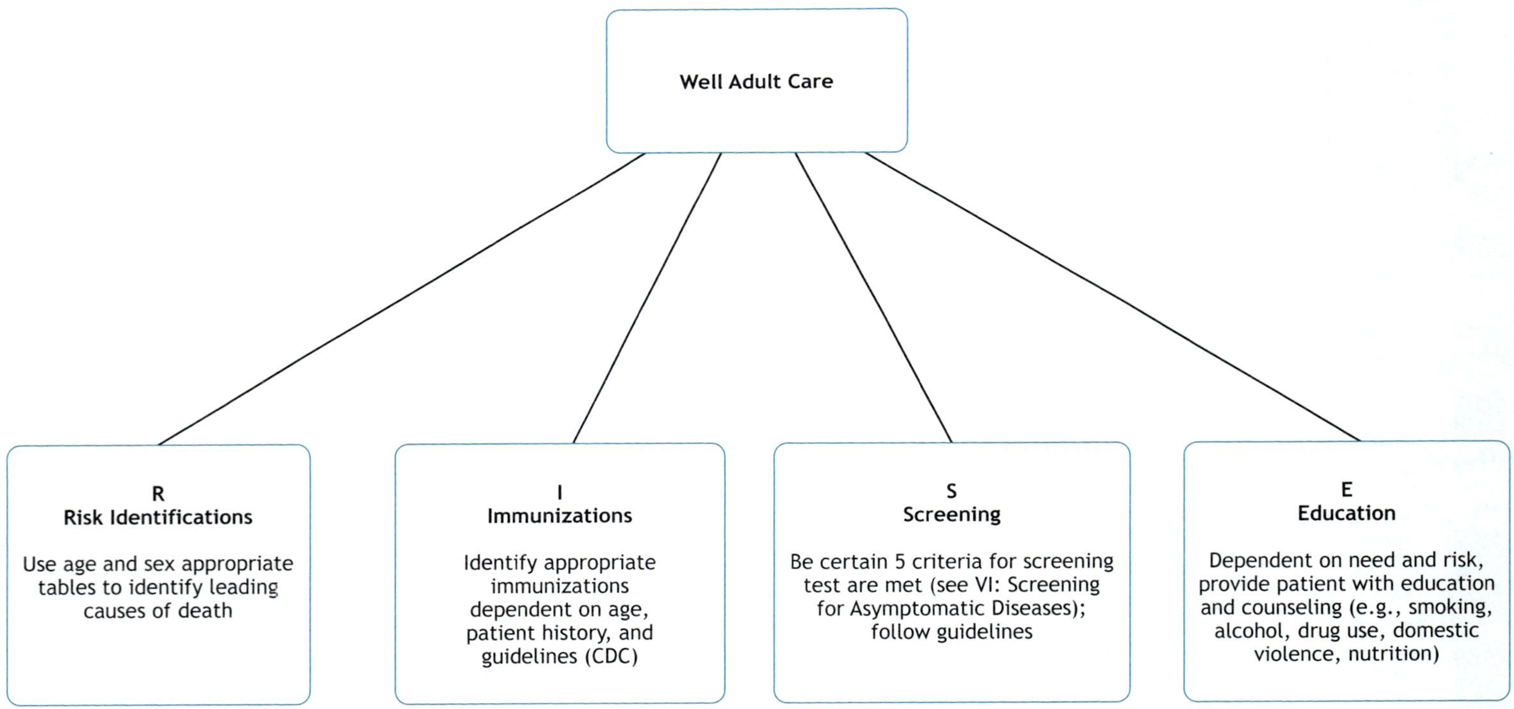

Figure 14–1. Well adult care visit using the RISE mnemonic.

Table 14–1. Death by etiology: all races, both males and females, all ages.

Rank	All races, both sexes, all ages	Number
	All causes	2,337,256
1	Diseases of the heart	724,859
2	Malignant neoplasm	541,532
3	Cerebrovascular disease	158,448
4	Chronic obstructive pulmonary disease	112,584
5	Accidents and adverse effects	97,835
6	Pneumonia and influenza	91,871
7	Diabetes mellitus	64,751
8	Suicide	30,575
9	Nephritis, nephritic syndrome	26,182
10	Chronic liver disease	25,192
	All other causes	463,427

Table 14–2. Death by etiology: all races, men aged 25–44 years.

Rank	All races, men aged 25–44 years	Number
	All causes	86,354
1	Accidents and adverse effects	20,232
2	Diseases of the heart	11,796
3	Suicide	9,700
4	Malignant neoplasm	9,684
5	HIV infection	6,509
6	Homicide and legal intervention	6,210
7	Chronic liver disease and cirrhosis	2,670
8	Cerebrovascular disease	1,703
9	Diabetes mellitus	1,507
10	Pneumonia and influenza	1,118
	All other causes	15,225

Table 14–3. Death by etiology: all races, men aged 45–64 years.

Rank	All races, men, aged 45–64 years	Number
	All causes	231,861
1	Malignant neoplasm	70,736
2	Diseases of the heart	70,138
3	Accidents and adverse effects	12,971
4	Cerebrovascular disease	8,466
5	Chronic liver disease and cirrhosis	8,031
6	Diabetes mellitus	7,139
7	Chronic obstructive lung disease	6,737
8	Suicide	6,201
9	Pneumonia and influenza	3,589
10	HIV infection	3,352
	All other causes	34,501

Table 14–4. Death by etiology: all races, men age 65 and older.

Rank	All races, men, age 65 and older	Number
	All causes	792,612
1	Diseases of the heart	270,637
2	Malignant neoplasm	199,794
3	Cerebrovascular disease	50,616
4	Chronic obstructive pulmonary disease	49,376
5	Pneumonia and influenza	35,790
6	Diabetes mellitus	20,862
7	Accidents and adverse effects	16,176
8	Nephritis, nephritic syndrome	10,533
9	Septicemia	7,687
10	Alzheimer's disease	6,913
	All other causes	124,228

Table 14–5. Death by etiology: all races, women aged 25–44 years.

Rank	All races, women, aged 25–44 years	Number
	All causes	45,028
1	Malignant neoplasm	11,723
2	Accidents and adverse events	6,940
3	Diseases of the heart	5,004
4	Suicide	2,502
5	HIV infection	2,149
6	Homicide and legal intervention	1,922
7	Cerebrovascular disease	1,617
8	Chronic liver disease	1,206
9	Diabetes mellitus	1,014
10	Pneumonia and influenza	813
	All other causes	10,138

Table 14–6. Death by etiology: all races, women aged 45–64 years.

Rank	All races, women, aged 45–64 years	Number
	All causes	148,342
1	Malignant neoplasm	62,035
2	Diseases of the heart	29,986
3	Cerebrovascular disease	6,940
4	Chronic obstructive pulmonary disease	6,253
5	Diabetes mellitus	5,952
6	Accidents and adverse effects	5,315
7	Chronic liver disease and cirrhosis	2,992
8	Pneumonia and influenza	2,434
9	Suicide	1,893
10	Septicemia	1,534
	All other causes	23,052

Table 14–7. Death by etiology: all races, women aged 65 years and older.

Rank	All races, women, 65 years and older	Number
	All causes	960,608
1	Disease of the heart	335,036
2	Malignant neoplasm	184,392
3	Cerebrovascular disease	88,528
4	Chronic obstructive pulmonary disease	48,520
5	Pneumonia and influenza	47,199
6	Diabetes mellitus	28,112
7	Accidents and adverse events	16,799
8	Alzheimer's disease	15,503
9	Nephritis, nephritic syndrome	12,107
10	Septicemia	11,325
	All other causes	173,087

Table 14–8. Well adult care recommendations for immunizations.

Immunization	Indications	Schedule	Contraindications/Special Concerns
Polio vaccine Inactivated vaccine (IPV) Oral (live) vaccine (OPV)	Routine adult vaccine not necessary Travelers to endemic areas Community members if outbreak Laboratory workers handling virus Health care workers at risk of exposure	Primary series is 3 doses	OPV not recommended in US Complete primary or incomplete series with IPV Select travelers should consider booster even if primary series is complete
Varicella vaccine	Absence of reliable history of disease Susceptible individuals at high risk		Avoid in cases of active tuberculosis, immunosuppression, immunodeficiency, pregnancy, recent immune globulin

(continued)

Table 14–8. Well adult care recommendations for immunizations. (continued)

Immunization	Indications	Schedule	Contraindications/Special Concerns
Hepatitis A vaccine	Travelers to endemic areas Men who have sex with men Illegal drug use Laboratory workers handling virus Chronic liver disease Clotting factor disorder	Two doses separated by 6–12 months	Avoid when hypersensitivity to alum or 2-phenoxyethanol Pregnancy class C

1. The **prevalence of the disease** and the **burden of suffering** caused by the disease must be high enough to justify widespread screening.
2. The **condition** must have an **asymptomatic period** when treatment will significantly reduce morbidity or mortality.
3. Acceptable **methods of treatment** must be available at **reasonable costs.**
4. The **screening test and interventions** must be **effective,** with few adverse effects.
5. The **screening test** must have **high sensitivity.**
   a. In some screening tests, there is a high likelihood of **false-positives,** which can lead to costly and more invasive procedures. Studies have shown that patients with a shorter life expectancy due to other illness or health status are less likely to benefit from screening.
   b. Table 14–9 summarizes recommendations for well adult screening tests.
   c. Table 14–10 summarizes recommendations for screening for cancer.

CLINICAL SKILLS TIP

If a screening test has a high false-positive, it will result in costly and more invasive procedures. Make certain the criteria for the use of a screening test in an asymptomatic person are met before using that test.

D. **Education:** Depending on need and risk, patients should be counseled on the following issues:
1. **Smoking:** If a patient smokes, advice should be given about smoking cessation programs, and the physician should follow up as necessary.
2. **Alcohol and drug abuse:** Counseling should be given concerning the dangers of driving under the influence of alcohol and drugs. Pregnant women should avoid all alcohol. Patients who are drug abusers should be offered counseling.
3. **Dental and oral health:** Patients should be advised to see a dentist regularly and brush and floss daily.
4. **Unintentional injury:** Patients should be taught about the importance of buckling seat belts when in moving vehicles and using safety equipment such as

Table 14–9. Recommendations for well adult care screening.

Screen	When to Begin	Interval	Tools/Special Concerns	Level of Evidence for Effectiveness
For Women				
Physician breast examination	Age 18	With mammogram or annually	Should not be used alone in place of mammogram	B/I
Self breast examination	Teach at visit when doing first Pap smear	Monthly	Efficacy questioned and not recommended by many groups Use to remind about mammograms	D/I
Chlamydia testing	When sexually active	Routine with Pap smear (annually) or other pelvic examinations until age 25 Women older than 25 at increased risk Pregnancy	Increased risk with multiple sexual partners, history of sexually transmitted diseases, or inconsistent condom use Cervical swab, self-administered vaginal swab, and urine tests being studied	A (first sexual activity to age 25) B (age > 25, high risk) C (age > 25, low risk)
For Men				
Prostate cancer testing: includes PSA testing and DRE	Aged 40–50 years	Unknown	Screening *not* recommended by most authorities	D
Chlamydia testing	First sexual activity	Periodically	Urethral swab and urine tests being studied	

Strength of Recommendations

The U.S. Preventive Services Task Force (USPSTF) grades its recommendations according to 1 of 5 classifications (A, B, C, D, I) reflecting the strength of evidence and magnitude of net benefit (benefits minus harms).

A.—The USPSTF strongly recommends that physicians provide [the service] to eligible patients. *The USPSTF found good evidence that [the service] improves important health outcomes and concludes that benefits substantially outweigh harms.*

(continued)

Table 14–9. Recommendations for well adult care screening. (continued)

Screen	When to Begin	Interval	Tools/Special Concerns	Level of Evidence for Effectiveness

B.—The USPSTF recommends that clinicians provide [this service] to eligible patients. *The USPSTF found at least fair evidence that [the service] improves important health outcomes and concludes that benefits outweigh harms.*

C.—The USPSTF makes no recommendation for or against routine provision of [the service]. *The USPSTF found at least fair evidence that [the service] can improve health outcomes but concludes that the balance of benefits and harms is too close to justify a general recommendation.*

D.—The USPSTF recommends against routinely providing [the service] to asymptomatic patients. *The USPSTF found at least fair evidence that [the service] is ineffective or that harms outweigh benefits.*

I.—The USPSTF concludes that the evidence is insufficient to recommend for or against routinely providing [the service]. *Evidence that the [service] is effective is lacking, of poor quality, or conflicting and the balance of benefits and harms cannot be determined.*

Table 14–10. USPSTF cancer screening recommendations.*

Cancer	Primary Prevention	Risk Factors	Secondary Preventions: Screening Recommendations	Comments
Breast	Low-fat diet	First-degree relative (premenopausal) (increase 2–3 fold): hx previous breast cancer, female, age; history of benign breast disease Some increased risk: 1st pregnancy >30 years Menarche <12 years Menopause after age 50; obesity, higher socioeconomic status, hx ovarian/endometrial cancer	Clinical breast exam: insufficient evidence Mammogram: aged 40–70 years every 1–2 years Breast self exam: easy, no cost involved, but insufficient evidence	28% of all newly diagnosed cancers in women 2nd highest death rate from cancer in women

(continued)

Table 14–10. USPSTF cancer screening recommendations.* (continued)

Cancer	Primary Prevention	Risk Factors	Secondary Preventions: Screening Recommendations	Comments
Colorectal	Low-fat high-fiber diet	First-degree relative; history of endometrial, ovarian, or breast cancer Inflammatory bowel disease (ulcerative colitis) Adenomatous polyps Colorectal cancer Familial polyposis coli	Fecal occult blood: age 50 and over yearly (3 samples) Sigmoidoscopy every 3 years after age 50 (+/- barium enema or colonoscopy)	Less than 10% of colorectal cancers palpable on rectal exam; 2nd most common cancer; Colonoscopy for high risk patients
Cervical	"Safe" sex, monogamy, abstinence	Low socioeconomic status History of multiple sexual partners Early onset of sexual intercourse (< 17 years) HPV; history of exposure to DES	Pap smear: Within 3 years of onset of sexual activity or at age 21, until age 65, every 2–3 years Do not do Pap smear after hysterectomy HPV testing: insufficient evidence	Stop at age 65 if other Pap smears all within normal range Pap smear: false - negative rate 80%
Skin	Limit sun exposure (clothing/hat/ sunscreen)	Sun exposure (sunburns); family history of melanoma and/or skin cancer; precursor lesions (dysplastic nevi, some congenital nevi)	No evidence for effective screening	Basal, squamous, malignant melanoma
Lung	Stop smoking; decrease exposure to second-hand smoke	Tobacco: over 90% etiology	No evidence for effective screening	Leading cause of cancer death
Prostate	??	??	No evidence for effective screening	Most common cancer in men; 3rd highest cancer mortality rate. Usually asymptomatic until metastatic

DES, diethylstilbestrol; HPV, human papillomavirus; USPSTF, United States Preventive Screening Task Force, 3rd edition. Courtesy of Judy Mello, MD, faculty, Scottsdale Family Practice Residency, Scottsdale, AZ.

helmets when riding motorcycles and bicycles; installing smoke detectors; and always having the telephone number of the poison control center available.

5. **Domestic violence:** Many patients will avoid discussing this topic, but it is important to offer counseling to those who have been or who are being abused.
6. **Nutrition:** Patients should be taught to maintain a healthy diet, as recommended by the United States Department of Agriculture and the United States Department of Health and Human Services.
   a. Eat a balanced diet.
   b. Balance diet with physical activity; maintain a suitable height/weight ratio.
   c. Eat plenty of whole grain products and vegetables and fruits.
   d. Maintain a diet low in fat (< 30% of calories), saturated fat (< 10% of calories), and cholesterol (≤ 300 mg per day).
   e. Choose a diet moderate in carbohydrates.
   f. Choose a diet moderate in sodium (< 2400 mg/day).
   g. Drink alcoholic beverages in moderation: no more than 1 drink per day for women, and no more than 2 drinks per day for men (1 drink = 12 oz of regular beer, or 5 oz of wine, or 1.5 oz of 80-proof distilled spirits).
7. **Physical activity:** Exercise is important, and patients should be educated about using caution in their exercise regimen; exercise should be gradual and enjoyable. Exercising at moderate intensity for ≥ 30 minutes about 5 days per week has proved to be sufficient.
8. **Sexually transmitted diseases, HIV, and unintended pregnancy:** Counseling should be tailored to the individual patient depending on risk, need, and ability.
9. **Skin cancer:** It is important to avoid excess sun exposure.

IV. **Special Cases:** Although there is insufficient evidence to recommend any particular preventive screening test, the United States Preventive Services Task Force (USPSTF) recommends that physicians be aware of

A. Skin lesions with malignant features
B. Peripheral arterial disease
C. Symptoms and signs of oral cancer, poor oral hygiene, and premalignant conditions
D. Subtle or nonspecific symptoms and signs of thyroid dysfunction
E. Changes in functional performance (with aging)
F. Depression
G. Suicide risk
H. Family violence
I. Drug abuse

V. **Challenges:** Adult well care and disease prevention are very important, but **it can sometimes be difficult to motivate either the patient or the physician.** Physicians are often poorly reimbursed for providing preventive care. Many adults, especially men, tend to avoid seeing the physician. This reluctance can add to the difficulty for the physician to provide this care.

CLINICAL CASE

A 47-year-old, otherwise well man comes to see you for a check-up. He tells you that he has been having a "midlife crisis" and that his family has suggested that he see a physician to make sure he is okay. He thinks he is going through the same things that his friends are experiencing: he is questioning his worth, his work, and his life. He feels fine physically. He denies any problems with sleep. His energy level is fine, and he remains interested in daily activities. He has continued to run 5 mornings every week with his friends. He completes work assignments and has no problems concentrating. His appetite is normal, and his weight has remained constant. He has not considered suicide. SIGECAPS are all negative (see Chapter 9). He has no significant past medical history and takes no medications. He has only been hospitalized once in his life, for a tonsillectomy as a child. Both of his parents are alive and in their 70s. He is not aware of any history of cancer in his family. He has not seen a physician for nearly 20 years and has had no blood tests or other studies performed, but he says many of his friends have seen their physicians recently and have had complete physicals and blood tests, so he thinks he should.

The reason this patient is seeing his physician is not uncommon—"make sure I'm okay, Doc." The physician has an ideal opportunity to engage this patient in healthy living practices and perform appropriate testing to help assure the patient that he is well. The patient mentions a "midlife crisis," and it is important that the physician ask appropriate questions regarding depression. Unfortunately, many physicians do not follow evidence-based guidelines, and many unnecessary tests are performed on patients like this gentleman. Using the RISE acronym (see III) can help guide the physician through this patient encounter.

Risk identification would indicate that the most likely cause of premature death for this 47-year-old gentleman would be due to accidents or adverse events. Cardiovascular diseases would be the second most likely cause of death in his age group. Our first effort (also the "E" in the acronym) should be focused on education. We want to counsel the patient about using seat belts and bicycle and motorcycle helmets, avoiding alcohol and driving, and providing general education regarding avoiding accidents.

Our patient has not seen a physician in nearly 20 years and has not received any **immunizations.** On further questioning, he is certain that he had chicken pox as a child. He should receive a tetanus booster. If he were to travel to endemic areas, we should counsel him about other immunizations that will be necessary.

A significant concern of this patient regards screening for asymptomatic disease. He tells you that his friends have all had multiple tests performed, and this is his expectation. At this time, it would be helpful to **provide him with some education regarding screening.** Another way of understanding the criteria used to justify a screening test is to divide the tests into disease criteria and test criteria. The **disease criteria** are

1. The disease must cause significant morbidity or mortality.
2. The disease must be common enough to justify screening.
3. Early detection and treatment must reduce morbidity or mortality (be cautious of lead-time bias: early diagnosis can appear to increase survival).

The **test criteria** are

1. The benefit of the test must outweigh the risk and the cost.

2. The test must be practical and feasible and acceptable to patients.
3. The test must be specific and sensitive enough to avoid large numbers of false-positives or false-negatives, respectively.

The last point regarding false-positives is often the most difficult to explain and convey to a patient. When the prevalence of a disease is extremely low, the likelihood of a false-positive result increases. **False-positives can lead to costly and more invasive procedures.** For example, in a young patient population where the prevalence of coronary artery disease is low, an exercise stress test will likely yield a false-positive result. This false-positive result will lead the physician to perform more tests, ultimately leading to the performance of a coronary angiogram. Acknowledging the low prevalence of disease in a population of young people should direct the physician and patient away from a screening test for coronary artery disease. Finally, some patients believe cost should not be an issue or concern. When told that national guidelines do not recommend the performance of an expensive test as a screening procedure, a patient may tell you that he/she has good insurance coverage and does not care about the cost. This is often a difficult discussion with a patient.

What should you do regarding the performance of tests to screen for asymptomatic disease? As noted above, there are many "authorities" and many "authoritative guidelines." As a physician, you should decide which guidelines you choose to follow and which to recommend. Guidelines from the USPSTF tell us that most authorities would not recommend screening for prostate cancer in our 47-year-old patient. Risk factors for colorectal cancer would include a first-degree relative who has colorectal cancer, inflammatory bowel disease (ulcerative colitis), or familial polyposis coli. The fecal occult blood test should be performed yearly beginning at age 50. Although there is evidence to recommend sigmoidoscopy, barium enema, or colonoscopy, most guidelines would recommend a complete colonoscopy at age 50 and, if normal, the procedure should be performed again in 10 years. Primary prevention should include counseling our patient to eat a low-fat, high-fiber diet. Other than stopping smoking or limiting exposure to second-hand smoke, there is no evidence for effective screening for lung cancer. The USPSTF recommends limiting sun exposure as primary prevention for skin cancer. Although there is no evidence for effective screening, patients with a family history of melanoma or skin cancer or those with precursor lesions such as dysplastic nevi should be examined regularly. **There is no consensus authoritative definition of "examined regularly."**

The last of the RISE acronym is **education.** Although difficult, lifestyle counseling can have a significant impact on a patient's health. Depending on need and risk, patients should be taught and provided with counseling on the issues noted in III D.

CLINICAL PEARLS

Patients will often ask and expect that numerous tests be ordered when they visit their physician. It is important to educate patients using evidence-based guidelines as to the appropriate use and lack of appropriate use of various tests and procedures.

CHAPTER 15

HYPERCHOLESTEROLEMIA

I. Defining Features

A. **Serum cholesterol in patients who have hypercholesterolemia is > 200 mg/dL (5.18 mmol/L).**

B. High-density lipoprotein (HDL) fraction of cholesterol is protective against heart disease.

C. Low-density lipoprotein (LDL) is atherogenic.

II. Epidemiology

A. In the United States, there are about 120 million people with a cholesterol level of ≥ 200 mg/dL and 60 million with a cholesterol level of ≥ 240mg/dL.

B. **More men than women have hypercholesterolemia;** prevalence increases with age.

C. About 2% of children, 20% of adult women, and 30% of adult men have elevated cholesterol levels.

III. Pathophysiology

A. Elevated cholesterol can result from single gene defects, polygenic disorders, or from the secondary effects of other disease states.

B. In the most common polygenic disorder, multiple genes interact with environmental factors to contribute to the hypercholesterolemia.

IV. Risk Factors

A. Obesity

B. Heredity

C. Sedentary lifestyle

D. Metabolic syndrome (Table 15–1)

V. Clinical Presentation

A. **Symptoms and History Related to Abnormalities of Cholesterol**

1. Angina pectoris
2. Claudication
3. Myocardial infarction (MI)
4. Stroke

Table 15-1. Metabolic syndrome: definition and treatment.

Metabolic syndrome is defined as any 3 of the following:	
Abdominal obesity	Defined by waist circumference, not BMI. Obesity is more closely associated with insulin resistance and the metabolic syndrome: Men > 102 cm (> 40 in) Women > 88 cm (> 35 in)
Triglycerides	≥ 150 mg/dL
HDL-C	Men < 40 mg/dL Women < 50 mg/dL
Blood pressure	≥ 130/≥ 85 mm Hg
Fasting glucose	≥ 110 mg/dL
Treatment is indicated if syndrome is present after 3 months of Therapeutic Lifestyle Changes (TLC)	
Underlying causes	Treat the underlying causes (overweight/obesity and physical inactivity): Intensify weight management Increase physical activity
Lipid and non-lipid risk factors	Treat lipid and non-lipid risk factors if they persist despite these lifestyle therapies: Treat hypertension Use aspirin for patients who have coronary heart disease to reduce prothrombotic state Treat elevated triglycerides and/or low HDL with pharmacotherapy

B. Signs Related to Abnormalities of Cholesterol

1. Corneal arcus before age 50
2. Xanthomata
3. Xanthelasma
4. Arterial bruits

CLINICAL SKILLS TIP

Xanthelasma and corneal arcus are physical findings that indicate a need to perform lipoprotein screening.

VI. Differential Diagnosis

A. Familial hypercholesterolemia

B. Polygenic hypercholesterolemia

C. Hypertriglyceridemia

1. Familial hypertriglyceridemia

2. Familial lipoprotein lipase deficiency
3. Familial apoprotein CII deficiency

D. Hypercholesterolemia with hypertriglyceridemia

E. Secondary causes of hyperlipoproteinemia
1. Diabetes mellitus (DM)
2. Hypothyroidism
3. Renal disease
4. Ethanol
5. Liver disease

RULE OUT

It is important to be alert to familial causes in which case other family members should also be screened.

VII. Diagnostic Findings

A. **Risk stratification regarding laboratory testing:** Lipid screening is followed by treatment using guidelines based on risk stratification developed by the National Heart, Lung, and Blood Institute (NHLBI), called the ATP III, which were updated in 2004 (Table 15–2). The three categories are

1. **Established coronary heart disease (CHD) and CHD risk equivalents:** CHD risk equivalents include noncoronary forms of clinical atherosclerotic

Table 15–2. Identified risk factors for hypercholesterolemia.*

Age	Men ≥ 45 years; women ≥ 55 years or those who have experienced premature menopause and are not taking HRT. CHD rates are higher in the elderly than in the young and are higher in men than in women of the same age.
Family history	A family history of premature CHD, defined as definite MI or sudden death ≤ 55 years in the father or a male primary relative, or ≤ 65 years in the mother or a female primary relative
Tobacco use	Men or women who currently smoke
Hypertension	Hypertension, defined as blood pressure > 140/90 mm Hg (confirmed by measurement on several occasions) or current use of any antihypertensive medication
Low HDL-C	Men or women who have a low HDL-C level (< 40 mg/dL)
"Negative risk"	HDL-C ≥ 60 mg/dL counts as a "negative" risk factor; its presence removes 1 risk factor from the total count

CHD, coronary heart disease; HRT, hormone replacement therapy; MI, myocardial infarction.
*Obesity and physical inactivity are not listed as risk factors, but should be considered as targets for intervention. Obesity is linked to other risk factors (eg, hypertension, hyperlipidemia, decreased HDL-C, and DM).

disease, DM, and multiple (2+) CHD risk factors with a 10-year CHD risk > 20%. The ATP III recommends that the Framingham risk scoring be carried out in individuals with 2+ risk factors to triage them into 3 levels of 10-year risk for high risk CHD events (MI and CHD death): > 20%, 10–20%, and < 10%. Therefore, patients with multiple CHD risk factors and a 10-year risk > 20% were elevated to the high-risk category. (The 10-year CHD risk can be calculated using a calculator found at the NHLBI web site referenced in the Appendix.)

2. **Multiple (2+) risk factors**
3. **Zero to one (0–1) risk factor**

B. Laboratory Studies

1. **Lipoprotein panel:** Total cholesterol, HDL, LDL, and triglycerides must be measured while fasting overnight (at least 9–12 hours).
2. Cholesterol is considered elevated if it is > 200 mg/dL (5.18 mmol/L).
3. Test **thyroid-stimulating hormone** (TSH) initially, because hypothyroidism may cause hypercholesterolemia.

Diagnostic Algorithm: see Figure 15–1: First Visit: Figure 15–2: Steps in Therapeutic Lifestyle Changes (TLC); Figure 15–3: Therapeutic approaches to persons with CHD or CHD risk equivalents; Figure 15–4: Therapeutic approaches to patients with multiple risk factors, 10-year risk 10–20%; Figure 15–5: Therapeutic approaches to the patient with multiple risk factors, 10-year risk <10%; Figure 15–6: Therapeutic approaches to persons with 0–1 risk factor.

VIII. Treatment (Figure 15–1; Tables 15–3 and 15–4)

A. The ATP III guidelines, revised in 2001, provide significantly greater direction regarding treatment goals than the previous guidelines. The **treatment depends on certain risk factors** (see Table 15–2).

B. Managing and maintaining a **balanced diet** is an important part of treatment.

1. The **therapeutic lifestyle change (TLC)** diet recommended by the ATP III states
   a. **Saturated fat intake** should be < 7% of calories, and cholesterol intake should be < 200 mg/day.
   b. **Increase intake of viscous (soluble) fiber (10–25 g/day) and plant stanols/sterols** (2 g/day) as therapeutic options to enhance reducing LDL.
2. **Eat a vegetarian-type diet,** with poultry, fish, and nonfat milk or yogurt, but **no eggs or cheese.**
3. A minimal intake of alcohol daily may increase HDL.
4. It is difficult to reduce cholesterol and weight if a diet is high in carbohydrates with a high glycemic index (eg, bread, rice, pasta, and potatoes).

C. Patients should be encouraged to **exercise** at least 2.5 hours per week. This can help them lose weight, decrease total cholesterol, and increase HDL.

D. Pharmacotherapy

1. **HMG-CoA Reductase Inhibitors (statins)**
   a. Fluvastatin (Lescol)
   b. Lovastatin (Mevacor)
   c. Pravastatin (Pravachol), Simvastatin (Zocor)

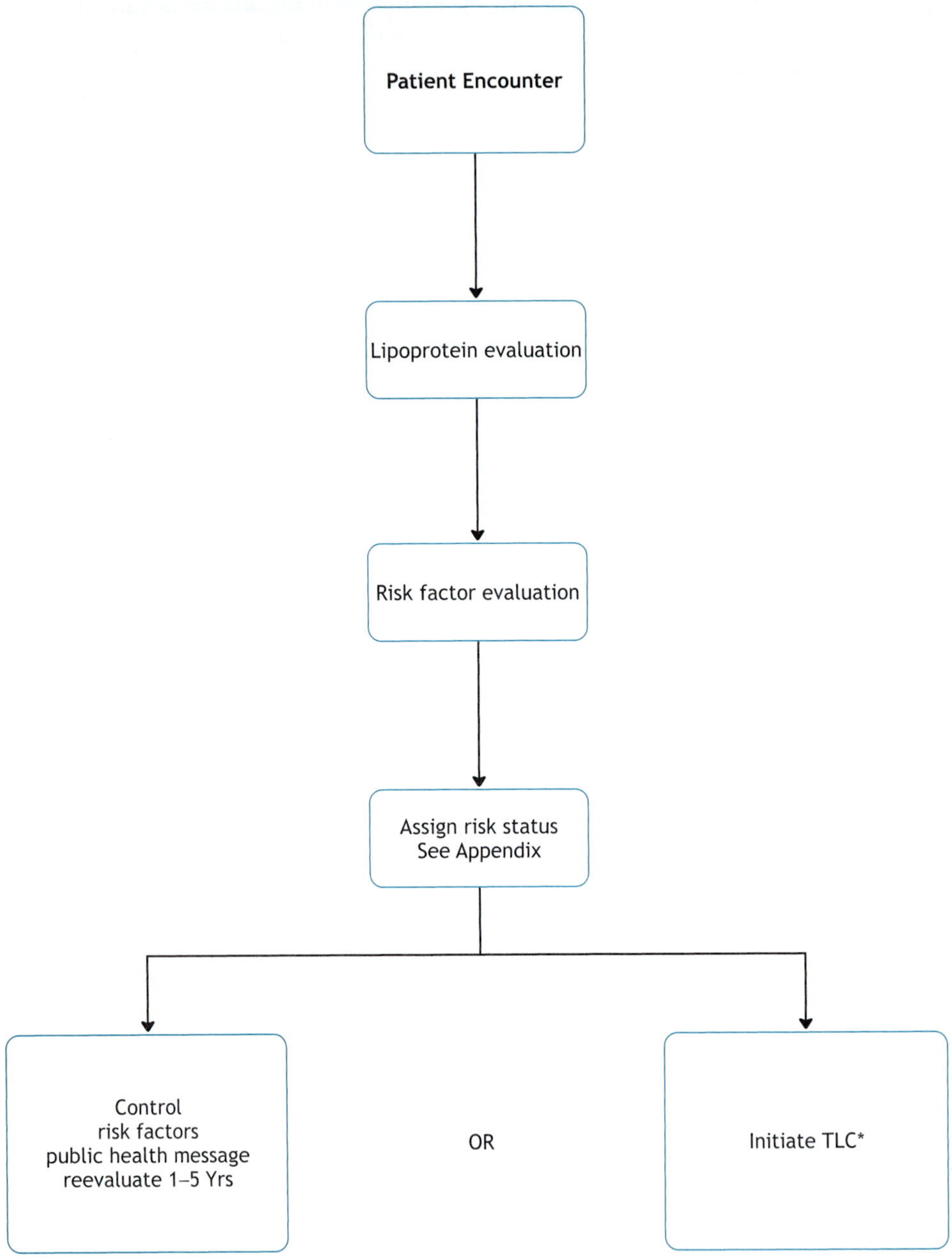

* If CHD or CHD-risk equivalent is present, drug therapy can be started simultaneously with TLC when LDL-C is ≥ 130 mg/dL.

Figure 15–1. First visit with the patient with hypercholesterolemia.

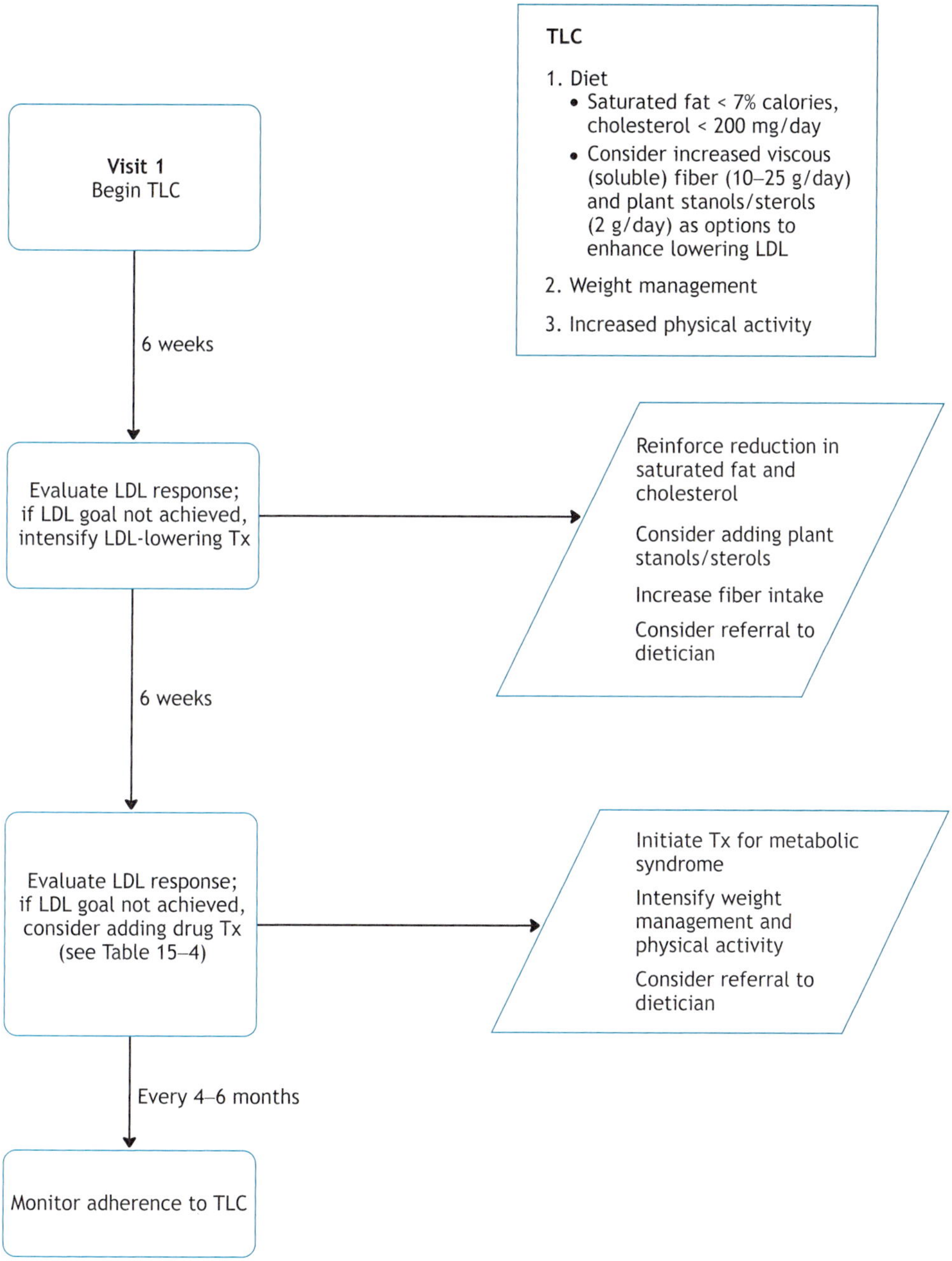

Figure 15–2. Steps in therapeutic lifestyle changes (TLC).

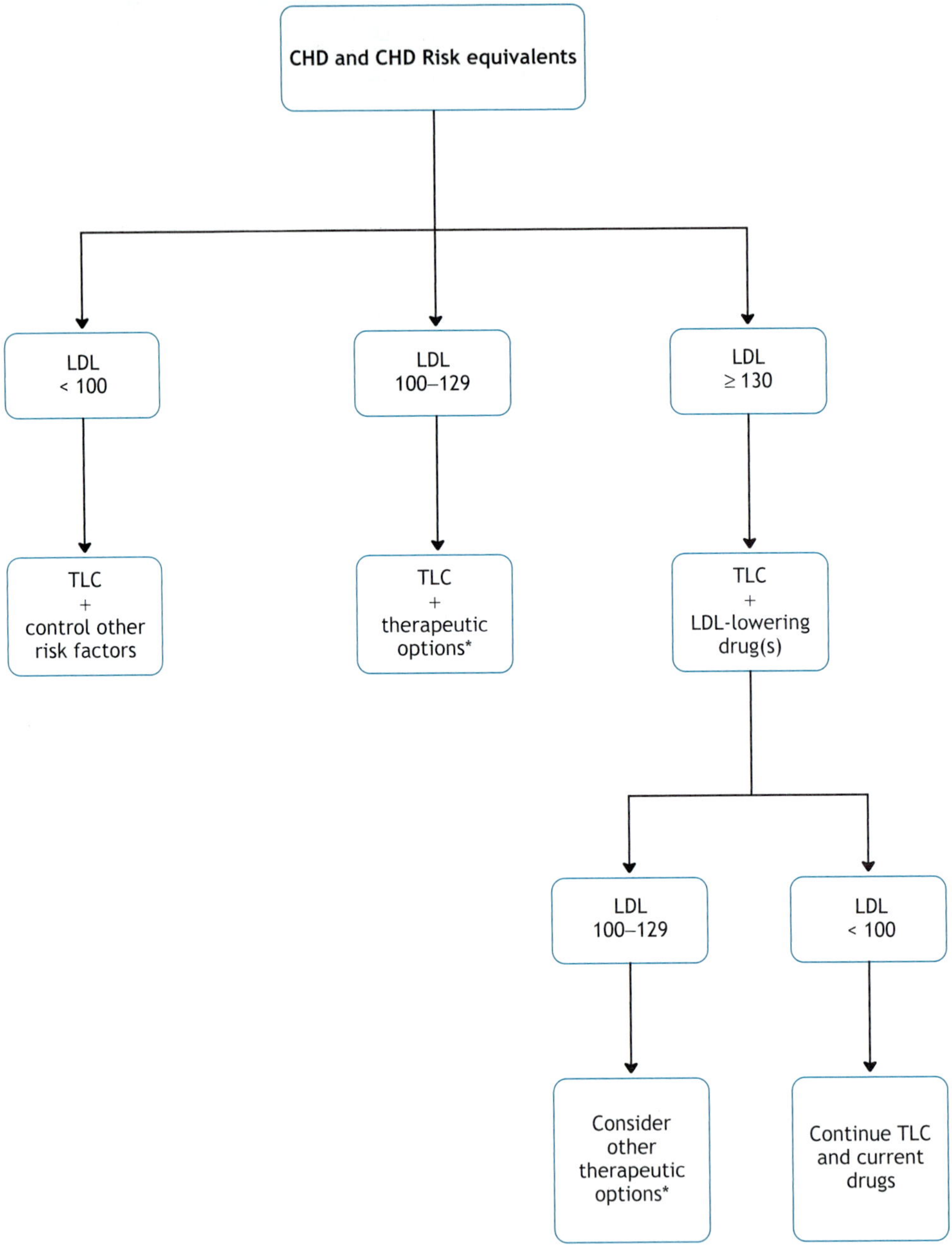

*Therapeutic options include intensifying LDL-lowering dietary or drug therapies, emphasizing weight reduction and increased physical activity, adding drugs to lower triglycerides or raise HDL (nicotinic acid or fibrates), and intensifying control of other risk factors.

Figure 15–3. Therapeutic approaches to the patient with coronary heart disease (CHD) or CHD risk equivalents (LDL-C goal is < 100 mg/dL).

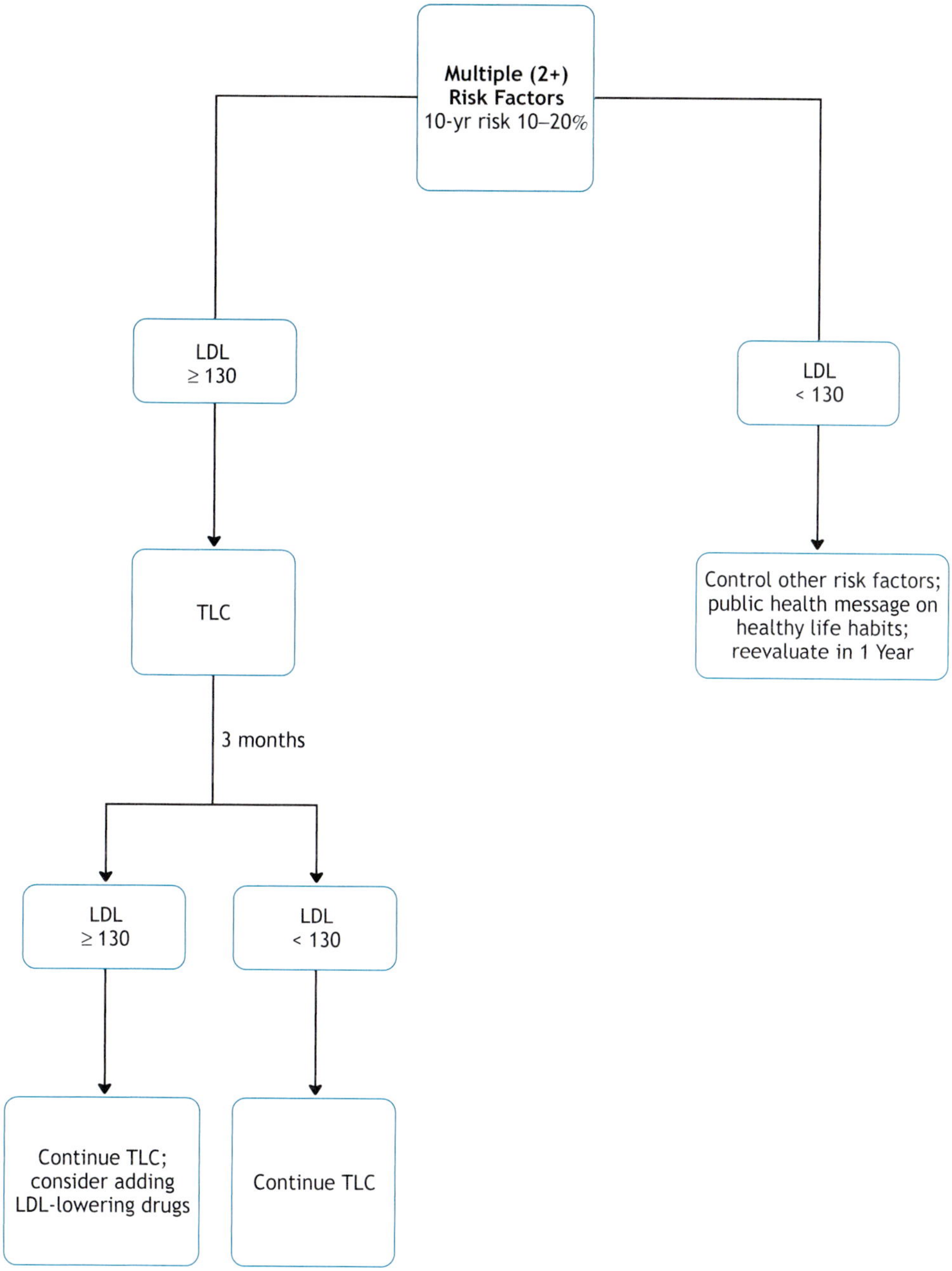

Figure 15–4. Therapeutic approaches to the patient with multiple risk factors, 10-year risk 10-20% (LDL-C goal is < 130 mg/dL. Drugs can be considered if necessary to attain LDL-C goal if the CLD-C level is ≥ 130 mg/dL after a trial of therapeutic lifestyle changes).

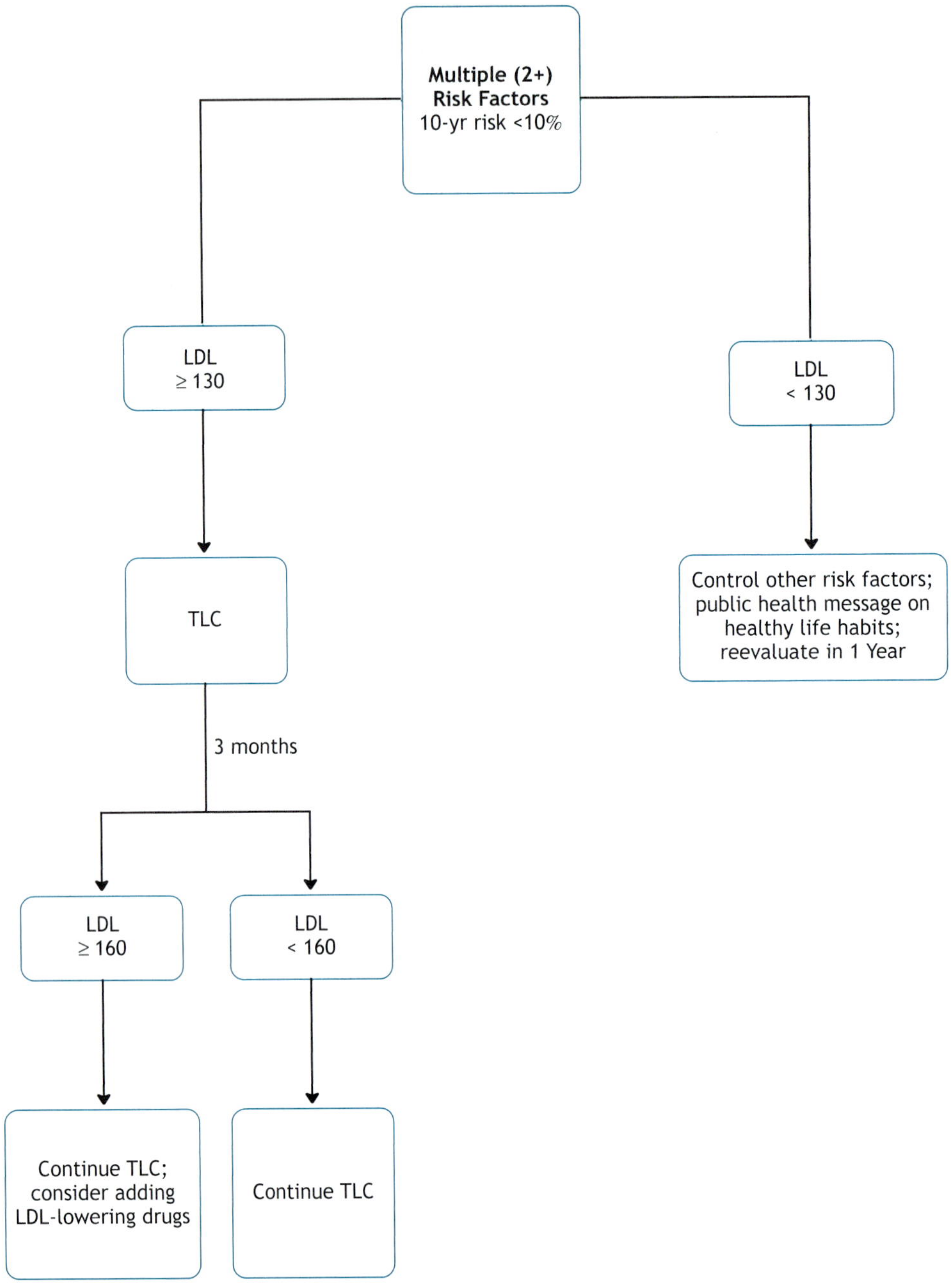

Figure 15–5. Therapeutic approaches to the patient with multiple risk factors, 10-year risk < 10% (LDL-C goal is < 130 mg/dL. Drug therapy can be considered if LDL-C is ≥ 160 after a trial of therapeutic lifestyle changes).

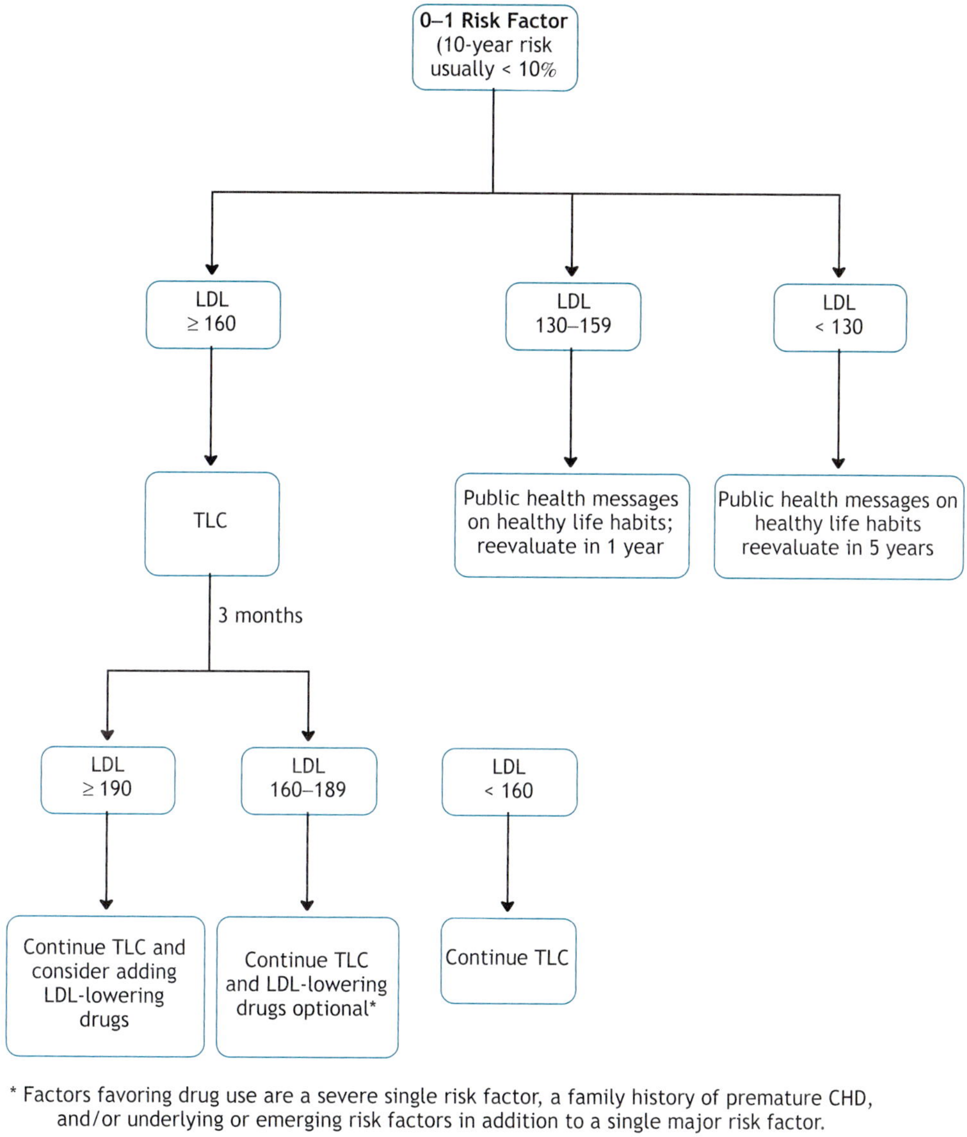

Figure 15–6. Therapeutic approaches to persons with 0–1 risk factor (The LDL-C goal is < 160 mg/dL. Drug therapy can be considered if the LDL-C level is ≥ 190 mg/dL after a trial of TLC. If LDL-C is 160–189 mg/dL, drug therapy is optional, depending on clinical judgment.)

Table 15–3. LDL cholesterol goals, therapeutic lifestyle changes (TLC), and drug therapy in different risk categories.

Risk category	LDL Goal	LDL Level at which to Initiate TLC	LDL Level at which to Consider Drug Therapy
CHD or CHD risk equivalents (10-year risk > 20%)	< 100 mg/dL	≥ 100 mg/dL	≥ 130 mg/dL (100–129 mg/dL: drug optional)*
2+ risk factors (10-year risk ≤ 20%)	< 130 mg/dL	≥ 130 mg/dL	10-year risk 10–20%: ≥ 130 mg/dL 10-year risk <10%: ≥ 160 mg/dL
0–1 risk factor†	< 160 mg/dL	≥ 160 mg/dL	≥ 190 mg/dL (160–189 mg/dL: LDL-lowering drug optional)

CHD, coronary heart disease.
* Some authorities recommend use of LDL-lowering drugs in this category if LDL-C < 100 mg/dL cannot be achieved by TLC. Others prefer use of drugs that primarily modify triglycerides and HDL (eg, nicotinic acid or fibrate). Clinical judgment also may call for deferring drug therapy in this subcategory.
† Almost all persons with 0–1 risk factor have a 10-year risk < 10%; thus 10-year risk assessment in people with 0–1 risk factor is not necessary.

Table 15–4. Drugs affecting lipoprotein metabolism.

Drug Class	Agents and Daily Doses	Lipid/Lipoprotein Effects	Side Effects	Contraindications
HMG-CoA reductase inhibitors (statins)	Lovastatin (20–80 mg), Pravastatin (20–40 mg), Simvastatin (20-80 mg), Fluvastatin (20–80 mg), Atorvastatin (10–80 mg), Cerivastatin (0.4–0.8 mg)	LDL-C ↓18-55% HDL-C ↑5-15% TG ↓7-30%	Myopathy Increased liver enzymes	**Absolute** • Active or chronic liver disease **Relative** • Concomitant use of certain drugs*

(continued)

Table 15–4. Drugs affecting lipoprotein metabolism. (continued)

Drug Class	Agents and Daily Doses	Lipid/Lipoprotein Effects	Side Effects	Contraindications
Bile acid sequestrants	Cholestyramine (4–16 g) Colestipol (5–20 g) Colesevelam (2.6-3.8 g)	LDL-C ↓15–30% HDL-C ↑3–5% TG No change or ↑	GI distress Constipation Decreased absorption of other drugs	**Absolute** • Dysbetalipoproteinemia • TG > 400 mg/dL **Relative** • TG > 200 mg/dL
Nicotinic acid	Immediate release (crystalline) nicotinic acid (1.5–3 gm), extended release nicotinic acid (Niaspan ®) (1–2 g), sustained-release nicotinic acid (1–2 g)	LDL-C ↓5–25% HDL-C ↑15–35% TG ↓20–50%	Flushing Hyperglycemia Hyperuricemia (or gout) Upper GI distress Hepatotoxicity	**Absolute** • Chronic liver disease • Severe gout **Relative** • Diabetes • Hyperuricemia • Peptic ulcer disease
Fibric acids	Gemfibrozil (600 mg BID) Fenofibrate (200 mg) Clofibrate (1000 mg BID)	LDL-C ↓5–20% (may be increased in patients with high TG) HDL-C ↑10–20% TG ↓20–50%	Dyspepsia Gallstones Myopathy	**Absolute** • Severe renal disease • Severe hepatic disease

GI, gastrointestinal; HDL-C, high-density lipoprotein cholesterol; LDL-C, low-density lipoprotein cholesterol; TG, triglycerides.

2. **Alternative Drugs**
   a. Cholestyramine
   b. Colestipol
   c. Niacin
   d. Ezetimibe

E. The ATP III guidelines were further updated in 2004. Since the publication of the ATP III, 5 major clinical trials of statin therapy with clinical end points have been published. These trials addressed issues that were not examined in previous clinical trials of cholesterol-lowering therapy. The trials added further support to the ATP III while leading the ATP III to make changes in 2004 (Table 15-5).

Table 15–5. Modifications to ATP-III treatment algorithm (2004).

New LDL-C goal	**I.** In high-risk persons, the recommended LDL-C goal is < 100 mg/dL; when risk is very high, an LDL-C goal of < 70 mg/dL is a therapeutic option (ie, a reasonable clinical strategy, on the basis of available clinical trial evidence). **II.** This therapeutic option also extends to patients at very high risk who have a baseline LDL-C < 100 mg/dL.
High TG or low HDL-C	When a high-risk patient has high triglycerides or low HDL-C, consider combining a fibrate or nicotinic acid with an LDL-lowering drug.
Moderately high risk persons	**I.** For moderately high-risk persons (2+ risk factors and 10-year risk 10–20%), the recommended LDL-C goal has been < 130 mg/dL, but an LDL-C goal < 100 mg/dL is a therapeutic option on the basis of these recent trials. **II.** A goal of LDL-C < 100 mg dL extends also to moderately high-risk persons with a baseline LDL-C of 100–129 mg/dL.
LDL-C percent reduction goal	When LDL-lowering drug therapy is employed in high-risk or moderately high-risk persons, it is advised that intensity of therapy be sufficient to achieve at least a 30–40% reduction in LDL-C levels.
TLC therapy	Any person at high risk or moderately high risk who has lifestyle-related risk factors (eg, obesity, physical inactivity, elevated triglycerides, low HDL-C, or metabolic syndrome) is a candidate for TLC to modify these risk factors regardless of LDL-C level.
Lower risk persons	For people in lower risk categories, recent clinical trials do not modify the goals and starting points of therapy.

CLINICAL CASE

A 43-year-old man comes to see you and says that he recently had his cholesterol tested at a health fair and that the results showed that his total cholesterol was 275 mg/dl and his HDL cholesterol was 30 mg/dL. He was told to see his physician to discuss the results. He currently has no health complaints. He has no past medical history other than ankle and femur fractures as a result of playing high school football. He takes no medications and has no allergies to medications. He has never been hospitalized. He is an only child and never knew his fa-

ther, who left the family when he was an infant. He learned through distant relatives that his father died in his early 40s, but no one knows the cause of his death, except that it was not an accident. The patient's mother is alive and is treated for type 2 DM. He is unaware of heart disease in his family. He is divorced and lives alone. Although he often tries to lose weight, he states that over the past 20 years since completing the university, he has progressively gained weight. He comments that he has tried many diets but none seem to work. Currently, he often eats fast food at work and at home. He stopped smoking 2 years ago and drinks about 1 six-pack of beer on the weekends. He does not use any illegal drugs. On physical examination, his vital signs show a blood pressure of 142/88 mm Hg, pulse is regular at 74, and his BMI is 27.5. HEENT, pulmonary, and cardiac examinations are normal. His abdominal examination reveals centripetal obesity but is otherwise unremarkable. His neurologic examination is non-focal.

This is a fairly common presentation of a patient who never sees a physician but receives a screening test at a local health fair and is referred to the office. This is an ideal opportunity to counsel this patient and engage him in health prevention practices. There are several issues to be addressed, beginning with the patient's **abnormal total cholesterol.**

National recommendations for cholesterol screening state that men older than age 34 and women older than age 44 should be screened every 5 years. The decision to screen men aged 20–34 years, women aged 20–44 years, and persons older than 75 years of age should be based on individual preferences of patient and provider. A complete lipid panel with cholesterol fractionation consisting of total cholesterol, HDL, LDL, and triglycerides should be measured, which requires that the patient fast from 9–12 hours. If it is unlikely that the patient will follow-up for the fasting blood test, one option is to check total and HDL cholesterol levels at the first visit, regardless of fasting. Although there are no clinical trials addressing the treatment of hyperlipidemia among men aged 20–34 years, women aged 20–44 years, or among men and women older than 75 years, screening based on nonlipid risk factors should be offered to patients in these age categories. For example, a 25-year-old man who has a primary relative whose total cholesterol is > 300 mg/dL or has a history of premature CHD should be screened.

By using these guidelines, we can **screen our patients, perform risk stratification, and begin appropriate lipid-lowering therapy** when appropriate. For our patient, we can conclude that if he had sought health care sooner and because of his family history, we would have discussed lipid screening with him beginning at age 20. At age 34, we would have advised him to have a complete lipid panel. Although the cause of his father's death is unknown, it is likely that he died of heart disease. If we do know that his death was not caused by an accident or trauma, statistics show that heart disease would be a likely cause. Therefore, **beginning at age 20, we could begin discussing lipid screening and, based on our patient's preference, perform the studies earlier than age 34.**

Next, we would **perform risk stratification** and would calculate his risk score as 8% (see Appendix). **This patient's 2 risk factors are low HDL and a family history of early cardiac death,** which would place him in the middle of the 3 risk categories. For a moderately high-risk person, the recommended LDL-C goal has been < 130 mg/dL, but an LDL-C goal of < 100 mg/dL is a therapeutic option based on the recent trials, discussed in VIII. The lower LDL-C goal would more likely apply to a patient whose 10-year risk score was 10–20% (our patient's is only 8%). If our patient were still smoking, or if he were 45 years of age, his risk score would be 10%, which would suggest an LDL-C goal of < 100mg/dL.

Our patient's **treatment would include both TLC and pharmacotherapy,** depending on the results of his LDL-C.

For most patients, **statins are the drugs of choice for lowering LDL-C,** and aggressive treatment with statins should be pursued. Statins also have a modest effect on reducing triglycerides and increasing HDL-cholesterol. Bile acid sequestrants, niacin, fibric acids, and ezetimibe can also be used. Niacin has a greater effect on reducing triglycerides and increasing HDL-C than do statins, but many people are intolerant of the side effects of niacin. The bile acid sequestrants are not systemically absorbed but may increase triglyceride levels. Fibric acids may be considered when both triglycerides and LDL-C are elevated or for an isolated low HDL-C. As monotherapy, ezetimibe has modest LDL-C lowering effects.

Monotherapy of patients with hypertriglyceridemia depends on their triglyceride levels. Patients with triglycerides > 500 mg/dL are at increased risk of developing acute pancreatitis. This risk increases significantly as triglycerides increase to > 1000 mg/dL. Fibric acids and niacin are the drugs of choice for these patients. Although triglycerides may not normalize with either drug, the risk of pancreatitis is reduced.

Some patients will require **combination therapy.** Most likely, these patients will have CHD. Low doses of 2 complementary agents, used concomitantly, can often reduce LDL-C to a greater extent than a higher dose of either agent alone, such as when a statin is combined with a bile acid sequestrant or ezetimibe, with fewer side effects and possibly less cost. In very resistant cases, triple therapy may be needed.

For patients who have **mixed hyperlipidemia** (increased LDL-C and triglycerides), the primary goal of decreasing LDL-C is the same as in patients with hypercholesterolemia alone. A high triglyceride level (200–499 mg/dL) with hypercholesterolemia signals a relatively high risk of CHD. These patients often have a low HDL-C. A **combination of a cholesterol-lowering drug with a triglyceride-lowering drug,** to achieve the non-HDL-C goal, may be most warranted in patients who have established coronary artery disease and who are at very high risk of recurrent coronary events. Combining nicotinic acid with a statin is favorable for improving levels of LDL-C, HDL-C, and triglycerides. Use of fibric acids can lead to an effective decrease in triglycerides and increased HDL-C, but their effect on LDL-cholesterol is varied (see Table 15–3).

CLINICAL PEARLS

Screen patients; follow ATP III guidelines; and be aggressive in managing their lipid levels.

CHAPTER 16
HYPERTENSION

I. Defining Features

A. Sustained elevated blood pressure (BP): **systolic BP ≥ 140 mm Hg** and/or **diastolic BP ≥ 90 mm Hg**

B. See Table 16–1 for further classification of hypertension.

II. Epidemiology

A. About 50 million people in the United States have elevated BP. Of these, 70% are aware of their diagnosis, but only 50% are receiving treatment; only 25% have their BP under control using a threshold criterion of 140/90 mm Hg.

B. **Onset of hypertension** usually occurs in persons in their **20s and 30s.**

C. In the United States, **hypertension affects 10–15% of white adults and 20–30% of African-American adults.**

D. Men are more likely to have hypertension than women.

III. Pathophysiology

A. Hypertension is characterized by **sympathetic nervous system hyperactivity.**

B. **Renin-antigiotensin system:** Renin is secreted by the juxtaglomerular cells surrounding afferent arterioles in response to a number of stimuli, including reduced renal perfusion pressure, diminished intravascular volume, circulating catecholamines, increased sympathetic nervous system activity, increased arteriolar stretch, and hypokalemia.

C. **Defect in natriuresis:** In hypertensive patients, there is a **diminished ability to excrete a sodium load.**

IV. Risk Factors

A. Cigarette smoking

B. Age (men older than age 55; women older than age 65)

C. Diabetes

D. Obesity

E. Excessive intake of alcohol

F. Dyslipidemia

G. Family history of cardiovascular disease, including hypertension and heart disease

Table 16–1. Classification of hypertension.

Classification	Systolic Blood Pressure	Diastolic Blood Pressure
Normal	< 120 mm Hg	< 80 mm Hg
Pre-hypertension	120–139 mm Hg	80–89 mm Hg
Stage 1 hypertension	140-159 mm Hg	90–99 mm Hg
Stage 2 hypertension	≥ 160 mm Hg	≥ 100 mm Hg

H. High dietary intake of caffeine and saturated fats

I. Stress

J. High sodium intake

V. Clinical Presentation

A. Symptoms of Hypertension

1. Hypertension should be considered **asymptomatic** except in extremes or after related cardiovascular complications develop.
2. **Headache,** often present **on awakening and occipital**, may occur, especially in patients who have a very high BP (> 220/120).

B. Signs of Hypertension

1. **Retinopathy:** narrowed arteries, atrioventricular (AV) nicking, copper or silver wiring of retinal arterioles.
2. **Increased second component of the aortic closure (A2) heart sound**
3. **Forceful precordial apical thrust**

CLINICAL SKILLS TIPS

- *When diagnosing hypertension, take 2 blood pressure readings 5 minutes apart, with the patient sitting in a chair. Confirm an elevated reading in the contralateral arm.*
- *Although the tension to compress the overlying tissues is usually regarded as negligible, a large circumference arm will yield readings 10–15 mm Hg higher than the actual pressure, unless a wide cuff (thigh cuff) is used.*

VI. Differential Diagnosis

A. Secondary Hypertension

1. Secondary hypertension is a differential diagnosis, but additional tests should be considered only if the history, physical, or basic laboratory evaluation indicates the possibility of this diagnosis.
2. There is a **low incidence of reversible secondary hypertension.**

B. Causes of Secondary Hypertension

1. **Chronic kidney disease:** Elevated creatinine or abnormal urinalysis
2. **Cushing's syndrome:** Truncal obesity, glucose intolerance, and purple striae

3. **Primary aldosteronism:** Unprovoked hypokalemia
4. **Renovascular disease:** Suspected with onset of hypertension before age 30, especially in the absence of family history, abdominal bruit, and accelerated hypertension; BP that has been easy to control but now is resistant; or acute renal failure precipitated by therapy with an angiotensin-converting enzyme (ACE) inhibitor or angiotensin receptor blocker.
5. **Pheochromocytoma:** Labile hypertension or paroxysms of hypertension accompanied by headache, palpitations, pallor, and perspiration.
6. **Coarctation of the aorta:** Decreased blood pressure in the lower extremities or delayed or absent femoral pulses.

RULE OUT

Secondary causes of hypertension include chronic kidney disease, primary aldosteronism, renovascular disease, pheochromocytoma, and coarctation of the aorta.

VII. Diagnostic Findings

A. Laboratory Studies

1. **Hemoglobin**
2. **Urinalysis and renal function studies:** Detect hematuria, proteinuria, and casts, signifying primary renal disease or nephrosclerosis.
3. **Serum-potassium level:** Determine if there is mineralocorticoid excess.
4. **Fasting blood sugar level:** Hyperglycemia occurs in patients who have diabetes mellitus (DM) and/or pheochromocytoma.
5. **Plasma lipids:** Indicator of atherosclerosis risk and additional target for therapy.
6. **Serum uric acid:** If elevated, relative contraindication to diuretic therapy.

B. Imaging Studies

1. **Electrocardiography:** The **"strain" pattern of ST-T wave changes** is a sign of more advanced disease and is associated with poor prognosis.
2. **Echocardiography** should be used to evaluate patients with clinical symptoms or signs of cardiac disease.

C. Diagnostic Procedures

1. Further diagnostic studies are indicated only if clinical presentation or routine tests suggest secondary or complicated hypertension.
2. Studies can include tests to determine endocrine causes of hypertension (24-hr urinary metanephrine); renal ultrasound to diagnose primary renal disease; and imaging studies to determine if there is renal artery stenosis.

VIII. Treatment

A. Treatment for Hypertension

1. Treatment s**hould begin upon assessment of overall cardiovascular risk** rather than by measurement of BP alone.
2. **Pharmacotherapy** should be prescribed for patients who have systolic blood pressure ≥ 140 mm Hg or diastolic blood pressure ≥ 90 mm HG. The goal for patients who have DM is BP ≤ 130/80 mm Hg.

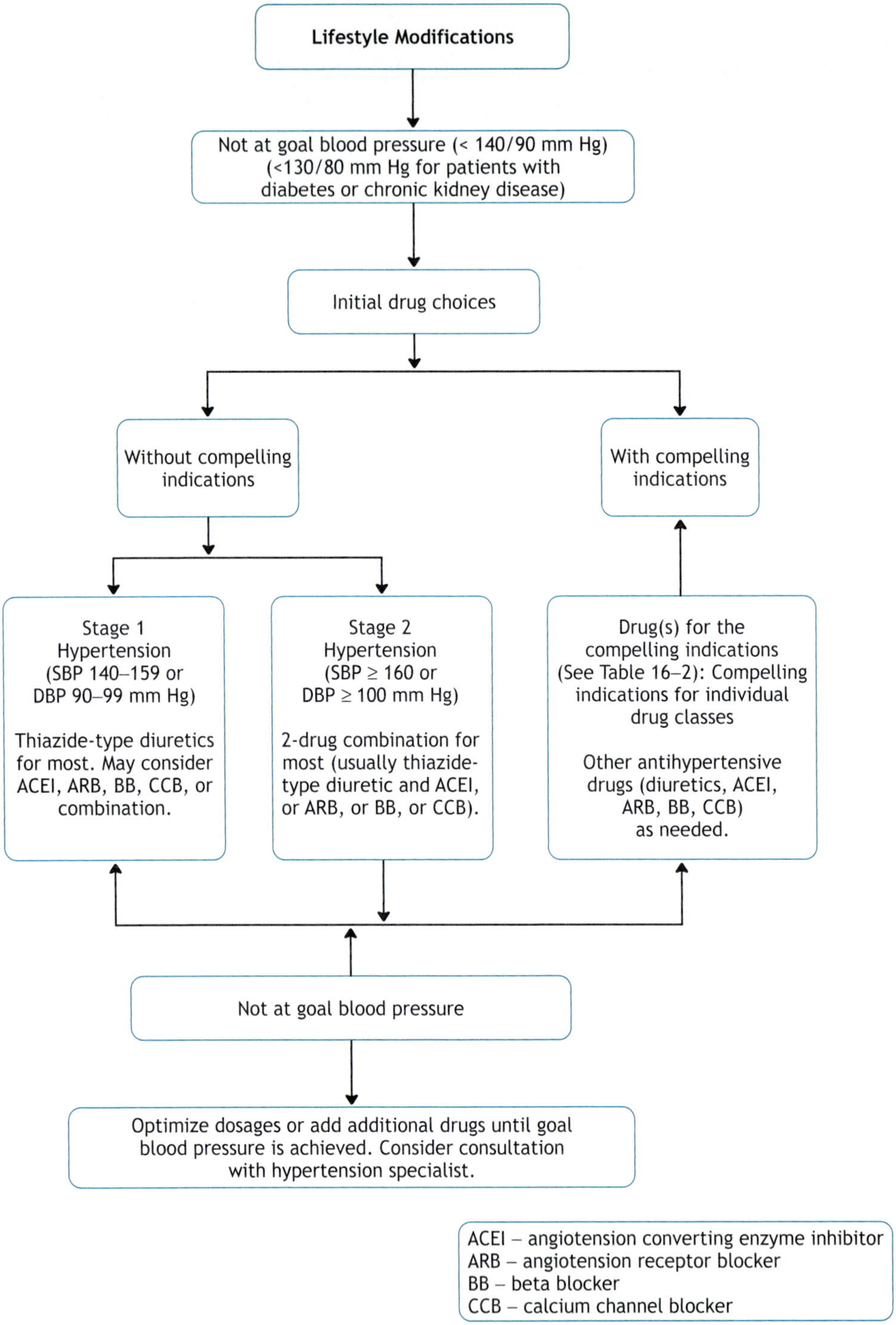

Figure 16–1. Algorithm for the treatment of the patient with hypertension. With permission from *http://www.nhlbi.nih.gov/guidelines/hypertension/jnc7full.htm.*

Table 16–2. Recommendations for lifestyle modification.

Modification	Recommendation	Average Systolic Blood Pressure Reduction Range
Weight reduction	Maintain normal body weight (BMI 18.5–24.9 kg/m^2)	5–20 mm Hg/10 kg
DASH eating plan	Adopt a diet rich in fruits, vegetables, and low-fat dairy products with reduced content of saturated and total fat	8–14 mm Hg
Dietary sodium reduction	Reduce dietary sodium intake to ≤ 100 mmol per day (2.4 g sodium or 6 g sodium chloride)	2–8 mm Hg
Aerobic physical activity	Regular aerobic physical activity (e.g., brisk walking) at least 30 minutes daily, most days of the week	4–9 mm Hg
Moderation of alcohol consumption	Men: limit ≤ 2 drinks per day. Women and lighter weight persons: limit ≤ 1 drink per day	2–4 mm Hg

B. **Lifestyle Modifications** (Figure 16–1; Table 16–2)
   1. Prescribe lifestyle modifications for **all patients who have been diagnosed with pre-hypertension or hypertension.**
   2. Components of lifestyle modifications include weight loss, DASH eating plan (**D**ietary **A**pproaches to **S**top **H**ypertension), dietary sodium reduction, aerobic physical activity, and moderation of alcohol consumption.

C. **Pharmacotherapy:** Almost all patients will require two medications to reach goal. Table16–3 summarizes oral hypertensive drugs by class, and Table 16–4 summarizes compelling indications for prescribing certain drugs.
   1. Diuretics
   2. β Adrenergic blocking agents
   3. β Blockers with intrinsic sympathomimetic activity
   4. Combined α and β blockers
   5. Angiotensin-converting enzyme (ACE) inhibitors
   6. Angiotensin II antagonists
   7. Calcium-channel blockers: nondihydropyridines
   8. Calcium-channel blockers: dihydropyridines
   9. α-Adrenoceptor antagonists: α-1 blockers
   10. Drugs with central sympatholytic action: central α-2 agonists
   11. Direct vasodilators

Table 16–3. Oral antihypertensive drugs*

Class	Drug (Trade Name)	Usual Dose Range in mg/Day	Usual Daily Frequency*
Thiazide diuretics	Chlorothiazide (Diuril)	125–500	1–2
	Chlorthalidone (generic)	12.5–25†	1
	Hydrochlorothiazide (Microzide, HydroDIURIL	12.5–50	1
	Polythiazide (Renese)	2–4	1
	Indapamide (Lozol†)	1.25–2.5	1
	Metolazone (Mykrox)	0.5–1.0	1
	Metolazone (Zaroxolyn)	2.5–5	1
Loop diuretics	Bumetanide (Bumex†)	0.5–2	2
	Furosemide (Lasix†)	20–80	2
	Torsemide (Demadex†)	2.5–10	1
Potassium-sparing diuretics	Amiloride (Midamor†)	5–10	1–2
	Triamterene (Dyrenium)	50–100	1–2
Aldosterone receptor blockers	Eplerenone (Inspra)	50–100	1
	Spironolactone (Aldactone†)	25–50	1
β-Blockers	Atenolol (Tenormin†)	25–100	1
	Betaxolol (Kerlone†)	5–20	1
	Bisoprolol (Zebeta†)	2.5–10	1
	Metoprolol (Lopressor†)	50–100	1–2
	Metoprolol extended release (Toprol XL)	50–100	1
	Nadolol (Corgard†)	40–120	1
	Propranolol (Inderal†)	40–160	2
	Propranolol long-acting (Inderal LA†)	60–180	1
	Timolol (Blocadren†)	20–40	2
β-Blockers with intrinsic sympathomimetic activity	Acebutolol (Sectral†)	200–800	2
	Penbutolol (Levatol)	10–40	1
	Pindolol (generic)	10–40	2
Combined α- and β-blockers	Carvedilol (Coreg)	12.5–50	2
	Labetalol (Normodyne, Trandate†)	200–800	2
ACE inhibitors	Benazepril (Lotensin†)	10–40	1
	Captopril (Capoten†)	25–100	2
	Enalapril (Vasotec†)	5–40	1–2
	Fosinopril (Monopril)	10–40	1
	Lisinopril (Prinivil, Zestril†)	10–40	1
	Moexipril (Univasc)	7.5–30	1
	Perindopril (Aceon)	4–8	1
	Quinapril (Accupril)	10–80	1
	Ramipril (Altace)	2.5–20	1
	Trandolapril (Mavik)	1–4	1

(continued)

Table 16–3. Oral antihypertensive drugs* (continued)

Class	Drug (Trade Name)	Usual Dose Range in mg/Day	Usual Daily Frequency*
Angiotensin II antagonists	Candesartan (Atacand)	8–32	1
	Eprosartan (Teveten)	400–800	1–2
	Irbesartan (Avapro)	150–300	1
	ILsartan (Cozaar)	25–100	1–2
	Olmesartan (Benicar)	20–40	1
	Telmisartan (Micardis)	20–80	1
	Valsartan (Diovan)	80–320	1–2
Calcium-channel blockers—nondihydropyridines	Diltiazem extended release (Cardizem CD, Dilacor XR, Tiazac†)	180–420	1
	Diltiazem extended release (Cardizem LA)	120–540	1
	Verapamil immediate release (Calan, Isoptin†)	80–320	2
	Verapamil long acting (Calan SR, Isoptin SR†)	120–480	1–2
	Verapamil (Coer, Covera HS, Verelan PM)	120–360	1
Calcium-channel blockers—dihydropyridines	Amlodipine (Norvasc)	2.5–10	1
	Felodipine (Plendil)	2.5–20	1
	Isradipine (DynaCirc CR)	2.5–10	2
	Nicardipine sustained-release (Cardene SR)	60–120	2
	Nifedipine long-acting (Adalat CC, Procardia XL)	30–60	1
	Nisoldipine (Sular)	10–40	1
α_1-Blockers	Doxazosin (Cardura)	1–16	1
	Prazosin (Minipress†)	2–20	2–3
	Terazosin (Hytrin)	1–20	1–2
Central α-2 agonists and other centrally acting drugs	Clonidine (Catapres†)	0.1–0.8	2
	Clonidine patch (Catapres-TTS)	0.1–0.3	1 wkly
	Methyldopa (Aldomet†)	250–1,000	2
	Reserpine (generic)	0.1–0.25	1
	Guanfacine (Tenex†)	0.5–2	1
Direct vasodilators	Hydralazine (Apresoline†)	25–100	2
	Minoxidil (Loniten†)	2.5–80	1–2

ACE inhibitors, angiotensin converting enzyme inhibitors.

* In some patients who are treated once a day, the antihypertensive effect may diminish toward the end of the dosing interval (trough effect).

Blood pressure (BP) should be measured just prior to dosing to determine if satisfactory BP control is obtained. Accordingly, an increase in dosage or frequency may need to be considered. These dosages may vary from those listed in the Physician's Desk Reference (57th ed.).

† Available now or becoming available soon in generic preparations.

Source: *Physician's Desk Reference,* 57th ed. Montvale, NJ: Thompson PDR, 2003.

Table 16–4. Compelling Indications for Individual Drug Classes

Compelling Indication	Initial Therapy Options
Heart failure	THIAZ, BB, ACEI, ARB, ALDO ANT
Post-myocardial infarction	BB, ACEI, ALDO ANT
High risk for cardiovascular disease	THIAZ, BB, ACEI, CCB
Diabetes	THIAZ, BB, ACEI, ARB, CCB
Chronic kidney disease	ACEI, ARB
Recurrent stroke prevention	THIAZ, ACEI

ACEI, angiotensin-converting enzyme inhibitor; ALDO ANT, aldosterone antagonist; ARB, angiotensin-receptor blocker; BB, β blocker; CCB, calcium-channel blocker; THIAZ, thiazide diuretic.

IX. Summary Table

Disease	Pathophysiology	Diagnostic Studies	Treatment
Primary hypertension	Sympathetic nervous system hyperactivity; defect in natriuresis	Urinalysis; K^+, uric acid; ECG, lipids	See Figure 16–1
Secondary hyper-tension: estrogen use	Volume expansion	None	Stop estrogen
Renal disease	Glomerular, tubular interstitial, polycystic kidneys	Urinalysis, creatine, BUN, renal ultrasound, abdominal CT	Control BP and comorbid conditions (eg, DM)
Renal vascular hypertension	Fibromuscular hyperplasia	Radioisotope renography, MRI or CT angiography; renal arteriography (gold standard)	Surgically correct lesion; treat hypertension
Primary hyperaldosteronism	Adrenal adenoma	K^+, abdominal CT scan or MRI	Correct lesion
Pheochromocytoma	Endocrine based	Urinalysis; abdominal CT scan or MRI	Correct lesion; treat hypertension
Coarctation of aorta	Obstruction	Angiography	Correct lesion

BP, blood pressure; BUN, blood urea nitrogen; CT, computerized tomography; DM, diabetes mellitus; ECG, electrocardiography; K^+, potassium; MRI, magnetic resonance imaging.

CLINICAL CASE

A 25-year-old man comes to see you after having his pre-employment physical. The examining physician found that his BP was 150/92 mm Hg and suggested that he follow-up with his regular physician. The patient has no complaints. He has no past medical history. Both of his parents have hypertension, but he does not know their ages at diagnosis. He smokes about 1 pack of cigarettes a day and drinks about 1 six-pack of beer on weekends. He does not use illegal drugs. On physical examination, his BP is 148/92 mm Hg in the right arm and 150/90 mm Hg in the left arm. His BMI is 30.5. Other vital signs are normal. His pulmonary and cardiac examinations are normal. No extra heart sounds or murmurs are heard. There is no bruit audible on his abdominal examination, and his kidneys are not palpable.

Hypertension rarely has presenting symptoms and is generally found on a routine physical examination. The United States Preventive Services Task Force (USPSTF) strongly recommends that physicians screen adults aged 18 and older for high blood pressure. There is good evidence that the blood pressure measurement can identify adults at increased risk for cardiovascular disease due to high blood pressure, and there is good evidence that treatment of high blood pressure substantially decreases the incidence of cardiovascular disease and causes little major harm.

When hypertension is identified in patients between the ages of 20 and 50, it is considered primary hypertension. Although there are multiple causes of secondary hypertension, **diagnostic testing would only be performed in certain situations,** including

1. All patients who have had **the initial diagnosis before the age of 20 or after the age of 50.**
2. Patients whose **hypertension** was previously well controlled, but it is **now refractory to treatment.**
3. Patients with an **epigastric or renal artery bruit.**
4. Patients where there is an **abrupt worsening of renal function after administering an ACE inhibitor.**
5. Patients with **hypokalemia (without diuretic therapy).**
6. Patients with **episodic sustained elevated BP.**

Other factors related to hypertension, particularly with this patient, are **obesity and alcohol use.** Weight loss and limiting alcohol use often can lead to normalization of the BP without medication.

CLINICAL PEARLS

Hypertension is generally asymptomatic; investigate for a secondary cause of hypertension in patients who are initially diagnosed before the age of 20 or after the age of 50.

CHAPTER 17

NORMAL PREGNANCY

I. Defining Features

A. Missed menses

B. Nearly any sign or symptom in a woman of child-bearing age

II. Epidemiology

A. The teenage pregnancy rate has decreased every year since 1991.

B. In 2002, pregnancy rates among females aged 15–19 was 43 births per 1000 females.

C. In 2002, pregnancy rates among women aged 35–44 years increased.

D. In 2002, about 84% of pregnant females received prenatal healthcare.

E. **The rate of infant, neonatal, and postneonatal deaths has decreased since 2002.**

F. In 2002, white women aged 25–29 years had the most pregnancies.

III. Pathophysiology: The **maintenance of pregnancy** is a complex process involving many steps.

A. **Implantation:** Apposition of the blastocyst, trophoblast invasion, and decidualization.

B. **Maternal recognition of pregnancy:** Rescue of corpus luteum, immunologic acceptance, and decidual quiescence.

C. **Maintenance of pregnancy:** Contain infection and myometrial quiescence.

D. **Endocrine function:** Maternal adaptation, mobilization of nutrients, and mammary development.

E. **Parturition:** Retreat from pregnancy maintenance.

IV. Risk Factors: The following factors need to be considered regarding **referral to a high-risk perinatologist.**

A. **Past OB/GYN history**

1. Prior preterm delivery (< 37 weeks)
2. Intrauterine fetal demise (IUFD): 10 weeks after cardiac activity
3. Prior cervical/uterine surgery
4. Prior preterm labor requiring hospital admission (eg, early cervical change)
5. Fetal anatomic abnormality (eg, open neural tube defects in prior infant or first-degree relative)
6. History of prior complicated pregnancy

B. Medical History

1. Pre-existing diabetes
2. Gestational diabetes
3. HIV
4. Chronic hypertension
5. Systemic disease requiring ongoing care (eg, severe asthma, lupus, or inflammatory bowel disease)
6. Current mental illness requiring pharmacotherapy
7. Cancer
8. Seizure disorders
9. Hematologic disorders
10. Recurrent urinary tract infections/stones

C. Psychosocial

1. Substance use disorders, including cigarette smoking
2. Eating disorders
3. Postpartum depression

D. Conditions in Current Pregnancy

1. Relative body mass index (BMI) < 16.5
2. Age (younger than age 16 or older than age 40 at delivery)
3. Vaginal bleeding

V. Clinical Presentation

A. Symptoms Consistent with Pregnancy

1. Nausea with or without vomiting
2. Urinary frequency, urgency, or dysuria
3. Fatigue
4. Perception of fetal movement

B. Signs Consistent with Pregnancy

1. Cessation of menses
2. Anatomical changes in the breasts (tenderness and enlargement)
3. Discoloration of the vaginal mucosa
4. Increased skin pigmentation and development of abdominal striae

CLINICAL SKILLS TIP

Cervical cyanosis (Chadwick sign), cervical softening, uterine softening (Hegar sign), and uterine enlargement are all associated with pregnancy.

VI. Differential Diagnosis

A. Myoma

1. Myomas **cause an enlarged uterus** and **can be confused with pregnancy.**
2. The uterus usually is very firm and irregular.

B. Contiguous but **extrauterine mass**

C. Hematometra

D. Ovarian tumor

RULE OUT

When caring for any woman of reproductive age with signs or symptoms of pregnancy, the physician must always ask him/herself, "Is she pregnant?"

VII. Diagnostic Tests

A. **Laboratory studies for diagnosis:** Urine or blood test for **elevated levels of hCG**

B. **Prenatal testing** includes
   1. **Urinalysis** and culture
   2. **Complete blood cell count (CBC)** with red blood cell indices
   3. Serologic test for **syphilis**
   4. **Rubella** antibody titer
   5. **Blood group, Rh type,** atypical antibody screening
   6. **HBsAg** evaluation
   7. **HIV** screening
   8. Cervical cultures for ***Neisseria gonorrhoeae*** and **Chlamydia**
   9. **Pap smear** of the cervix
   10. **Sickle cell screening** for all African-American women; **hemoglobin electrophoresis** to identify abnormal hemoglobins in women of African, Asian, or Mediterranean ancestry with anemia or low MCV values.
   11. **Tuberculosis skin testing** for women who are immigrants or who live in inner cities.
   12. **Genetic counseling** with the option of chorionic villus sampling or genetic amniocentesis for **all women over age 35 years** and those who have prior offspring with chromosomal abnormalities.
   13. **Tay-Sachs** blood screening for Jewish women of European descent with Jewish partners of European descent.
   14. Screening for **cystic fibrosis**
   15. Screen women at high risk of **hepatitis C** infection with Hep C antibody.

C. **Prenatal Care (Table 17–1)**
   1. Pregnancy is measured in weeks from the start of the last menstrual period. A **normal full term pregnancy is 37–40 weeks.**
   2. By convention, a pregnancy is divided into **trimesters**. The first trimester ends at about 12 weeks; the second ends at about 24 weeks; and the third trimester ends with delivery.
   3. **Prenatal care** is described by **services delivered at visits, weeks, or by trimesters**. Table 17–1 describes the care delivered by week and visit.

D. **Not recommended:** There is inadequate evidence to recommend the following interventions during pregnancy:
   1. Antenatal pelvimetry
   2. Routine urine dipstick test
   3. Routine edema evaluation
   4. Screening for cytomegalovirus (CMV)
   5. Screening for bacterial vaginosis
   6. Vitamin supplementation
   7. Immunizations: measles, mumps, rubella (MMR) (recommendation in Table 17–1 refers only to preconception visit)

Table 17–1. Prenatal care by week of visit.

Visit	Screening Maneuvers	Counseling and Education	Immunizations and Chemoprophylaxis	Physical Examination	Laboratory Studies
All visits	—	Breast-feeding Exercise during pregnancy	—	Blood pressure	—
Preconception visit	Risk profiles Domestic abuse	Substance use Nutrition and weight Physical activity Violence and abuse Sexual practices Preterm labor prevention List of medications, herbal supplements, and vitamins Accurate recording of menstrual dates	Td booster MMR Varicella Hepatitis B Nutritional supplements	Height, weight, BMI Blood pressure Breast exam Abdominal & pelvic exam	Cholesterol and HDL Pap smear
Visit 1* 6–8 weeks (with OB intake nurse)	Self-questionnaire of prenatal risk factors*** Tobacco, alcohol, drug use Domestic violence	** Lifestyle Nutrition Warning signs of pregnancy loss Course of care Physiology of pregnancy Testing for risks in pregnancy	Td booster**** Varicella**** Hepatitis B**** Nutritional supplements		ABO Rh blood typing and antibody screen RPR Asymptomatic bacteriuria (urine culture) HIV Glucola, if indicated from history of gestational diabetes mellitus

(continued)

Table 17–1. Prenatal care by week of visit. (continued)

Visit	Screening Maneuvers	Counseling and Education	Immunizations and Chemoprophylaxis	Physical Examination	Laboratory Studies
Visit 2 **10–12 weeks** (with physician, midwife or nurse practitioner)	Weight Blood pressure Fetal heart tones	Fetal growth Review lab results Breast-feeding Body mechanics		Selected systems physical exam based on history Complete pelvic exam	Pap smear**** Gonorrhea & chlamydia CBC
Visit 3 **16–18 weeks**	Weight Blood pressure	Second trimester growth Quickening Lifestyle Physiology of pregnancy		Fetal heart tones Fundal height	OB ultrasound Maternal serum AFP screen (triple screen)
Visit 4 **22 weeks**	Weight Blood pressure	Preterm labor signs Class Family issues Length of stay Gestational diabetes mellitus RhoGAM		Fetal heart tones Fundal height	
Visit 5 **28 weeks**	Preterm labor risk Weight Blood pressure Domestic abuse screening	Work Physiology of pregnancy Preregistration Fetal growth Awareness of fetal movement Preterm labor symptoms	ABO/Rh/Ab (RhoGAM) if indicated Influenza	Fetal heart tones Fundal height Examine cervix	50 gm Glucola for gestational diabetes mellitus Rh antibody status

Visit 6 **32 weeks**	Weight Blood pressure Fetal movement counts	Travel Sexuality Pediatric care Episiotomy Labor and delivery issues Warning signs/PIH	Fetal heart tones Fundal height	
Visit 7 **36 weeks**	Weight Blood pressure Fetal movement counts	Postpartum care Management of late pregnancy symptoms Contraception When to call provider Discussion of post-partum depression	Fetal heart tones Fundal height Examine cervix Confirm fetal position	Culture for Group B streptococcus
Visits 8–11 **38–41 weeks**	Weight Blood pressure Fetal movement counts	Postpartum vaccinations Infant CPR Post-term management Labor and delivery update	Fetal heart tones Fundal height Examine cervix	Post-dates antenatal fetal testing

AFP, α-fetoprotein; BMI, body mass index; CBC, complete blood cell count; CPR, cardiopulmonary resuscitation; HDL, high-density lipoprotein; HIV, human immunodeficiency virus; MMR, measles/mumps/rubella; OB, obstetric; PIH, pregnancy-induced hypertension; RPR, rapid plasma reagin; Td, tetanus-diphtheria.

*It is acceptable that the history, physical, and laboratory studies listed under Visit 1 be deferred until Visit 2 if both the patient and the provider agree.

** Should also include all subjects listed for the preconception visit if none occurred.

***To be completed within 2 weeks of provider knowledge of pregnancy.

****If not done at preconception visit.

VIII. Treatment

A. **Early detection** of pregnancy is important so a wanted pregnancy can begin with prenatal care; women with unwanted pregnancies can be counseled about adoption or termination of the pregnancy.

B. Pregnant women should **begin prenatal care early** and schedule regular visits with the physician (or obstetrician).

C. Pregnant women should eat a **balanced diet** with fresh fruits and vegetables; take prenatal vitamins with iron and folic acid; decrease caffeine intake; avoid eating raw or rare meat; and always wash hands after handing raw meat.

D. Pregnant women should **stop drinking alcohol and taking illicit drugs** (these substances can affect the fetus).

IX. Summary Table

Condition	Pathophysiology	Diagnostic Studies	Treatment
Pregnancy	See III	Urine or serum hCG, pelvic ultrasound	Regular prenatal care
Myoma	Benign tumor of uterus resulting from estrogen stimulation	Endometrial biopsy, endovaginal ultrasound, hysteroscopy	Surgical or medical hormonal
Hematometra	Collection of blood and other menstrual fluid within the uterus causes uterusto distend	Pelvic ultrasound	Surgical
Ovarian tumor	Various etiologies leading to enlargement of the ovary	Pelvic ultrasound	Surgical or chemotherapy

CLINICAL CASE

A 23-year-old woman comes to see you because she is concerned that she is pregnant. She states that her last menstrual period was 4 weeks ago and that she took a home pregnancy test and it was positive. She otherwise feels fine. She has no children but has been pregnant twice previously. The first pregnancy was electively terminated, and the second pregnancy was terminated by miscarriage. She has no other significant past medical history and does not take any medications. She says that as a child she used to take medications for asthma, but has not used these for nearly 10 years. She was once taken to the emergency department for what was thought to be a seizure. She had an extensive work-up but was discharged without a diagnosis. She does not have diabetes mellitus, hypertension, or HIV infection. She says that she was tested for HIV 3 months ago before she began her current relationship. She has had

6 lifetime sexual partners but has no risk factors for HIV infection. As an early adolescent, she was thought to have an eating disorder, but her weight has been stable for the past 6 years. She does not use tobacco but has an occasional "joint" on the weekends. She drinks about 1 six-pack of beer on the weekends. She uses no illegal drugs. She is not worried about domestic violence and feels that she has a good relationship with her boyfriend (with whom she is pregnant). Her mother and maternal grandmother have type 2 diabetes mellitus, but there is no other significant family history. On physical examination, she appears happy and in no distress. Her vital signs reveal a blood pressure of 104/74 mm Hg and a BMI of 19.6. Findings from HEENT, cardiac, and pulmonary examinations are normal. Her abdomen is soft without masses. Pelvic examination reveals an anteverted uterus and no abnormal masses. The cervix is minimally red without discharge. Examination of the extremities is also within normal limits.

This patient presents with a relatively common complaint to a family physician's office. Because of the widespread availability of home pregnancy tests and their reasonable accuracy, many women perform a test before they have missed a menstrual period. The accuracy of home urine pregnancy tests is outstanding, with sensitivity as low as 20 mIU/mL/hCG. The physician can confirm the result in the office with a urine pregnancy test and then begin one of the most important parts of this woman's care: prenatal care. Although many family physicians no longer provide complete maternity care, including delivery, many will continue to provide prenatal care. By doing this, they are able to maintain their relationship with their patients and are prepared to provide clinical care for the newborn. **There are multiple sets of guidelines for prenatal care organized around recommended activities at each visit based on weeks' gestation.** These guidelines comment on issues such as tests, procedures, and educational activities. This section will focus on evidence-based activities that are recommended and discouraged for discussion at each prenatal visit. In many physicians' offices, the initial pregnancy-related visit is with a nurse. The patient completes a self-questionnaire, which is reviewed by the nurse with the patient assessing for risk factors that would suggest the need for referral or consultation (see Table 17–1). The family physician must determine if there are any indications for referral (see IV).

CLINICAL PEARLS

There are evidence-based national guidelines for prenatal care, and it is important to follow them. Some physicians may choose to perform activities that are no longer evidence-based, as noted in VII D.

CHAPTER 18
OSTEOARTHRITIS

I. Defining Features

A. Osteoarthritis occurs **most often secondary to other articular disease.**

B. It is characterized as a **degenerative disorder** without systemic manifestations.

C. **Pain** from osteoarthritis is usually **relieved by rest.** Morning stiffness is brief, and articular inflammation is minimal.

D. **Radiographic findings** show narrowed joint space, osteophytes, increased density of subchondral bone, and bony cysts.

II. Epidemiology

A. At least 20 million adults in the United States suffer from the effects of osteoarthritis.

B. This disease is the **most common form of joint disease.**

C. Osteoarthritis affects people of all ages, races, genders, and geographic areas.

D. It is the **leading cause of disability for persons older than age 65.**

III. Pathophysiology

A. Osteoarthritis is an arthropathy characterized by **degeneration of cartilage** and by **hypertrophy of bones at the articular margins.**

B. **Steps in Pathologic Change**

1. The articular cartilage is first **roughened** and finally worn away.
2. **Spur formation and lipping** occur at the edge of the joint surface.
3. The synovial membrane becomes **thickened, with hypertrophy** of the villous processes.
4. The joint cavity **never becomes totally obliterated**, and the synovial membrane does not form adhesions.

IV. Risk Factors

A. **Obesity** is a risk factor for developing osteoarthritis in the knee and most likely the hip.

B. Competitive **contact sports** also increase the risk of osteoarthritis.

C. Activities that require **frequent bending and carrying** increase the risk of osteoarthritis in the knee.

D. **Injury to a joint** is also a risk factor.

V. Clinical Presentation

A. Symptoms of Osteoarthritis

1. **Slowly developing joint pain.**
2. **Pain following use of a joint.**
3. **Stiffness** (especially in the morning and after sitting) of < 30 minutes duration.
4. Long-standing **pain that increases with weight bearing or walking upstairs and lessens with rest.**
5. In osteoarthritis of the spine, there is **local pain and stiffness with radicular pain** (if there is compression of nerve roots).

B. Signs of Osteoarthritis

1. **Joint enlargement** (eg, Heberden's nodes of distal interphalangeal joints and Bouchard of the proximal interphalangeal joints)
2. **Decreased range of motion (ROM)**
3. **Bony deformity** (osteophyte)
4. **Tenderness usually absent;** may be associated with synovitis, with tenderness along joint margin.
5. **Effusions are not warm** (as would occur in inflammatory or infectious arthritis).
6. **Crepitation** (late sign)

CLINICAL SKILLS TIP

Symptoms correlate poorly with the objective extent of joint disease. Heberden and Bouchard nodes are frequently encountered.

VI. Differential Diagnosis

A. **Degenerative joint disease** is easily distinguished from arthritis, because articular inflammation is minimal and systemic manifestations are absent.

B. To help **differentiate osteoarthritis from rheumatoid arthritis,** the physician should observe the distribution of joint involvement in the hands (distal vs proximal).

RULE OUT

The physician must rule out rheumatoid arthritis, an inflammatory joint disease that requires different treatment including use of DMARDs (disease modifying anti-rheumatic drugs).

VII. Diagnostic Findings

A. **Laboratory studies:** Elevated sedimentation rate and other laboratory signs of inflammation are not present.

B. Imaging Studies

1. **Radiographs** may reveal narrowing of the joint space, sharpened articular margins, osteophyte formation and lipping of marginal bone, and thickened, dense subchondral bone. Bone cysts may also be present.
2. For patients with knee pain, a **45° flexion weight-bearing posteroanterior plain radiograph** should be done.

C. Diagnostic Procedures: Joint Aspiration

1. It may be helpful to distinguish between osteoarthritis and chronic inflammatory arthritides.
2. In **osteoarthritis,** the cell count is usually < 500 cells/mm^3, predominantly mononuclear cells.
3. In **inflammatory arthritis,** the cell count is usually > 2000 cells/mm^3, predominantly neutrophils.

VIII. Treatment (Figures 18–1 and 18–2)

A. For patients who have **mild to moderate osteoarthritis of weight-bearing joints,** a **supervised walking program** may be helpful. **Weight loss** can also improve symptoms.

B. Total hip replacement provides excellent symptomatic and functional improvement when that joint is seriously afflicted. **Knee replacement** is effective, but arthroscopic surgery for knee osteoarthritis has proved ineffective.

C. Pharmacotherapy

1. Patients with mild osteoarthritis should take **acetaminophen** for pain management.
2. **Topical capsaicin cream** may be helpful to relieve pain in the hand or knee.
3. **Nonsteroidal anti-inflammatory drugs (NSAIDs)** should be used for patients who do not respond to acetaminophen.
4. **Tramadol** can be considered for those patients whose symptoms are not relived with NSAIDs.
5. **Intraarticular glucocorticoids** can provide symptom relief but can cause cartilage breakdown and should not be used frequently.
6. **Intra-articular hyaluronan** is indicated for patients who do not respond to nonpharmacologic therapy and analgesics.
7. **Glucosamine and chondroitin** have demonstrated some degree of efficacy.

IX. Summary Table

Condition	Pathophysiology	Diagnostic Studies	Treatment
Osteoarthritis of knee	Degradation of cartilage and hypertrophy of bones at articular margins	X-ray, including standing view	Acetaminophen; NSAIDs
Ligamentous injury	Sprain or strain	X-ray; MRI	Ice; knee immobilizer; non-weight bearing; possible surgery
Meniscal tear	Tear of meniscus	Clinical (eg, thorough knee examination) and MRI	NSAIDs; rest; surgery may be necessary
Patellofemoral syndrome	Overuse	Clinical and skyline x-ray views of knee	Rest; orthotics; stretching and muscle strengthening

(continued)

Summary Table (continued)

Condition	Pathophysiology	Diagnostic Studies	Treatment
Inflammatory arthritis	Inflammatory	Serologies; ESR; arthrocentesis	NSAIDs; DMARDs
Infectious arthritis	Local or hematogenous spread of infectious organism	CBC; ESR; arthrocentesis	Antibiotics
Osteoarthritis of hip	Degradation of cartilage and hypertrophy of bones at articular margins	X-rays	Acetaminophen; NSAIDs; see VIII C
Trochanteric bursitis	Often traumatic	Clinical diagnosis	NSAIDs; stretching
Iliotibial band syndrome	Overuse	Clinical diagnosis	NSAIDs; orthotics

CBC, complete blood cell count; DMARDs, disease modifying anti-rheumatic drugs; ESR, erythrocyte sedimentation rate; NSAIDs, nonsteroidal anti-inflammatory drugs.

CLINICAL CASE

A 72-year-old man comes to your office complaining of knee pain. Although he has experienced the pain for about 4 years, it has become significantly worse in the past week after he fell down the stairs and injured his left knee cap. Previously, the pain was present although tolerable. It began insidiously and has slowly increased over the past few years. The pain is dull and increases with most activity, but improves with rest. The patient points deep to his knee cap when asked where the pain is located. He says that ibuprofen and acetaminophen were somewhat helpful before this recent fall, but now the pain is more significant and constant. His prior history is significant for hypertension, angina, and diabetes mellitus, which are all controlled with oral medications of lisinopril, diltiazem, metoprolol, metformin, and glyburide. He has no surgical history, although he had multiple injuries to both knees while playing football in high school and college. He has continuously gained weight since his mid 30s. He is always on a diet, but has not been successful at losing weight. He used to play golf but stopped about 4 years ago, because the pain in his knees increased when walking around the golf course. He does not use tobacco. He has a glass of wine with dinner every night. On physical examination, his vital signs are within normal limits. His BMI is 33.5. Direct examination of his knees reveals swelling of both knees, more so in the left knee than the right; effusion with minimal ballottement; minimal synovial thickening; slight warmth; and minimal atrophy of the surrounding muscles. Active and passive ROM is restricted by about 10°. There is crepitus, pain, and muscle spasm at the extremes of existing ROM. There is no obvious joint deformity. Distal pulses are intact and symmetrical. Ex-

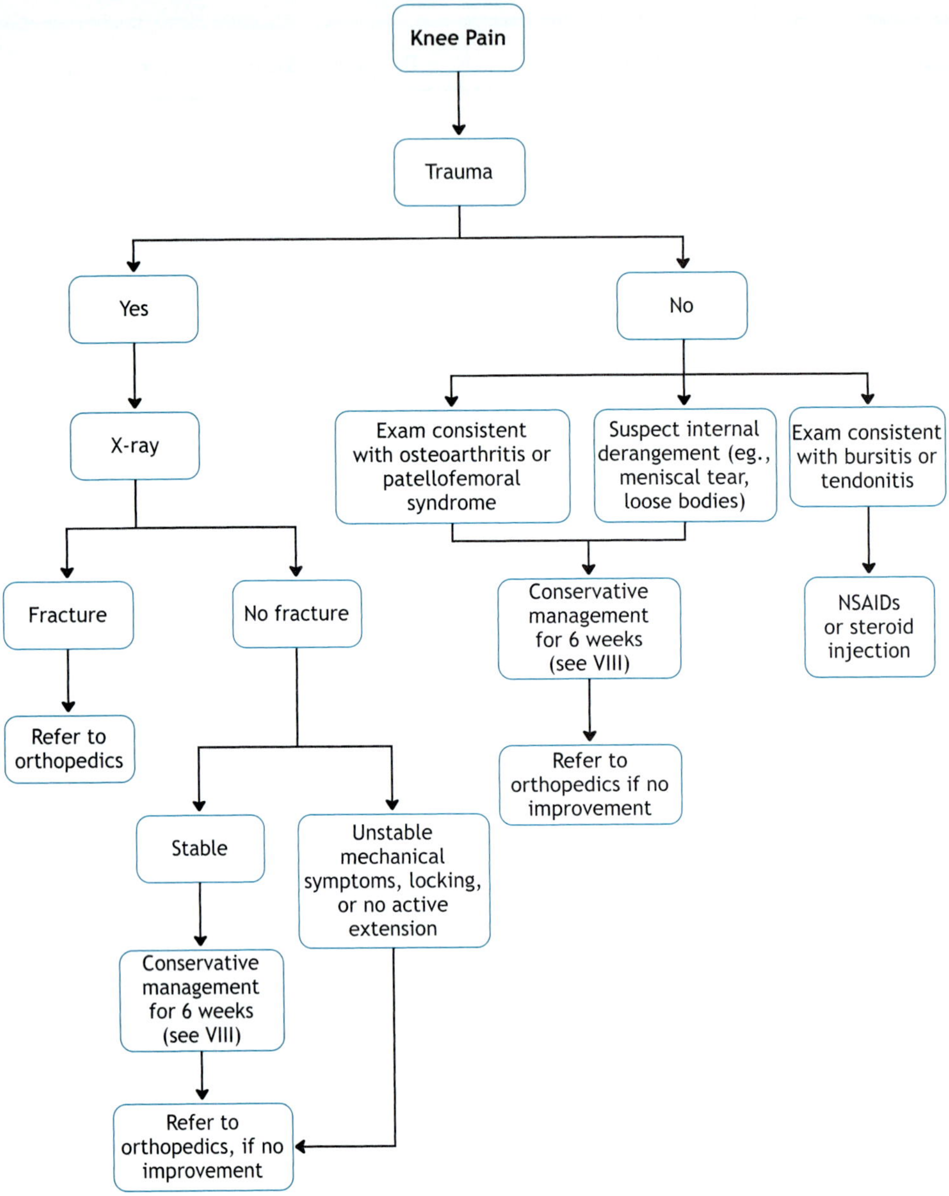

Figure 18–1. Management of the patient with knee pain.

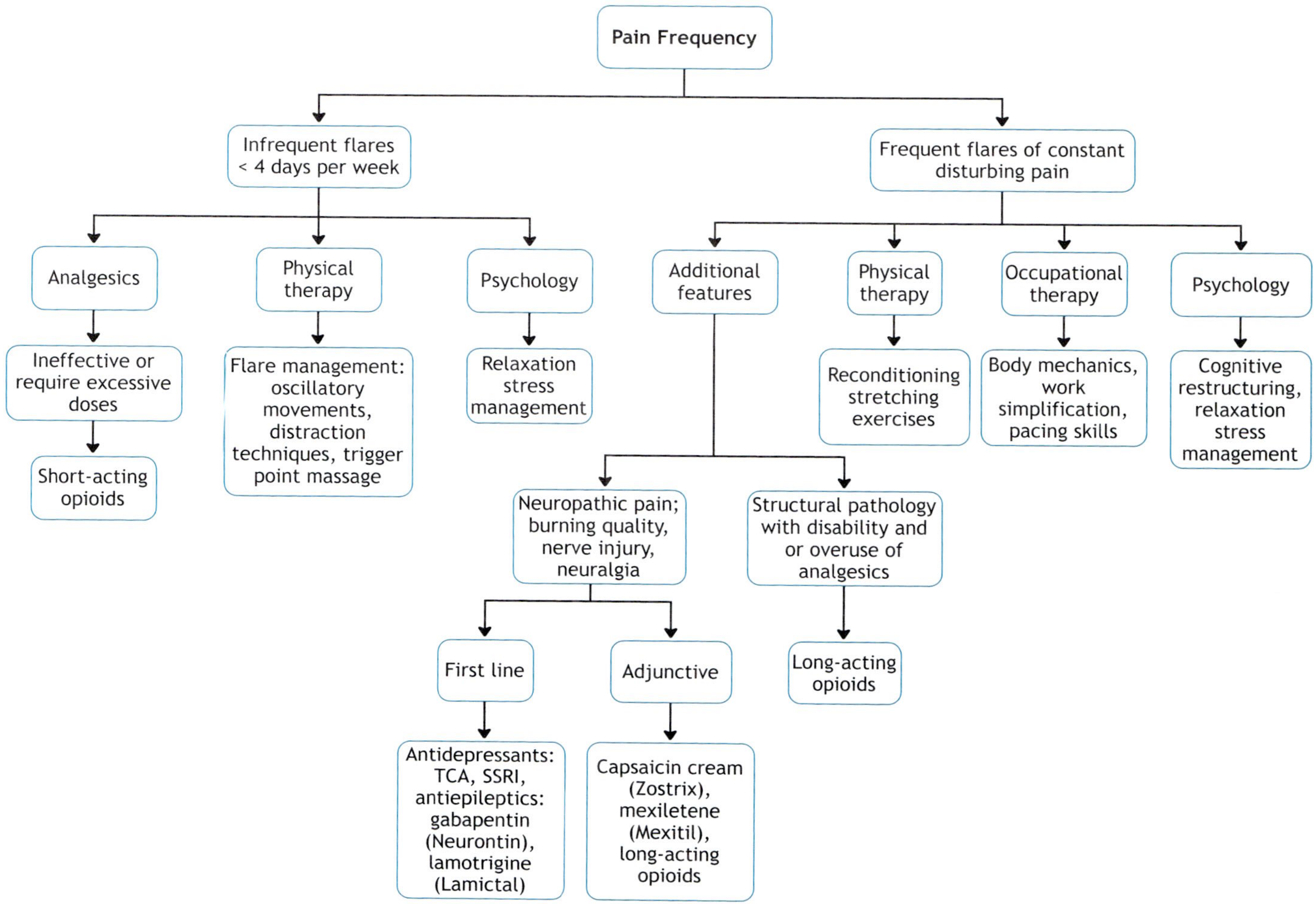

Figure 18–2. Management of the patient with chronic pain.

amination of the hips reveals minimal decrease in active ROM (5°). There is no crepitus and no pain.

This patient has osteoarthritis (also called degenerative joint disease) of his knees. Osteoarthritis is the most common form of joint disease and is an increasingly common problem in an increasingly elderly population. A history of prior knee injuries as well as obesity is associated with osteoarthritis. Our patient has many of the findings consistent with osteoarthritis (see V).

The physician must differentiate the pain associated with osteoarthritis from the pain that is caused by inflammatory arthritides, infectious arthritis, or traumatic injuries such as a meniscal tear. **The following signs and symptoms are not consistent with osteoarthritis:**

1. Fever or chills (infectious)
2. Erythema (infectious)
3. Warmth (infectious or inflammatory)
4. Large effusions (inflammatory)
5. Locking or giving away on examination of the knee (as would occur with a meniscal tear)

When a patient presents with any of the above signs and symptoms, the investigation should be directed to include serologies and erythrocyte sedimentation rate (ESR) (inflammatory); complete blood cell count (CBC) and arthrocentesis (infectious or inflammatory including gout); and imaging (meniscal tear). Each of these problems requires different and often more urgent treatment. If these symptoms are present, other diagnoses must be ruled out.

The next consideration by the physician relates to diagnostic work-up. **Indications for x-rays in the evaluation of joint pain include**

1. History of trauma to rule out fracture.
2. Presence of significant effusion, especially monarticular arthritis.
3. After physical examination, the pain cannot be explained by ligamentous strain or bursitis, and the patient has not had a prior x-ray of the joint.
4. There is loss of joint ROM without an established pre-existing condition.
5. The patient has severe joint pain, even with known pre-existing diagnosis of the joint.
6. Persistent significant knee pain, especially in a young patient.
7. Conservative treatment failed.
8. Referral to an orthopedist, if surgery is contemplated.

Laboratory studies would be completed if there were a nontraumatic effusion to rule out infectious or inflammatory arthritides. The fluid should be sent to the laboratory for Gram staining and culture, crystal analysis, and cell count and differential. It is not necessary to measure glucose and protein.

Treatment should include patient education, pain management, exercise, physical therapy, and assistive devices (such as walkers and canes) in certain situations. Patient education should include counseling regarding weight loss and self-management resources to learn activities and exercises that will benefit the condition. Physical and occupational therapists can instruct the patient in carrying out exercises, muscle strengthening, and

ROM activities. They may recommend wearing different footwear or orthotics; applying either ice packs or ice massage every 3–4 hours for a period of 15–20 minutes; or taking warm baths, using a heat lamp, heating pad, or warm compresses for 15–20 minutes. See VIII C for a discussion of options for pharmacologic therapy.

CLINICAL PEARLS

Osteoarthritis is common and presents with long-standing, insidious pain in the large joints.

CHAPTER 19
SMOKING CESSATION

I. Defining Features

A. The patient uses tobacco.

B. The patient expresses a willingness to stop smoking.

II. Epidemiology

A. **Cigarette smoking causes the most preventable deaths and early mortality.**

B. In 2000, an estimated 4.83 million premature deaths were attributed to cigarette smoking. Of these deaths, 2.41 million were in developing countries and 2.43 million were in industrialized countries.

C. **In 2000, more than three fourths of deaths attributed to cigarette smoking occurred in men.**

D. Smoking can result in cardiovascular, pulmonary, musculoskeletal diseases and cancers, which can all lead to premature death (Table 19–1).

E. In the United States, **23% of adults smoke;** 90% of adult smokers are addicted to nicotine.

F. **About 45% of adults attempt to quit smoking annually;** at least 70% have tried to quit at least once. **About 4% of smokers are able to quit each year.**

G. **Smokers die an average of 5–8 years earlier than persons who have never smoked.**

H. Smoking cessation reduces the risk of disease and can add years to a person's life. On average, women who quit smoking by age 35 add about 3 years to their life expectancy, and men add more than 2 years.

I. Smokers whose physicians advise them to quit smoking are 1.6 times more likely to attempt to quit.

III. Pathophysiology

A. **Nicotine increases the level of dopamine in the brain.**

B. **Discontinuation** of nicotine **produces withdrawal symptoms.**

IV. Risk Factors (see Table 19–1)

V. Clinical Presentation

A. Smokers may have **elevated blood pressure.**

B. They often have nicotine stains on their fingers and nails.

Table 19–1. Diseases associated with tobacco use.

System/Other	Associated Disease
Cardiovascular	Coronary artery disease including myocardial infarction Hypertension CVA
Pulmonary	Chronic obstructive pulmonary disease Chronic bronchitis Emphysema Invasive pneumococcal disease Lung cancer
Ear, nose, and throat	Mouth cancer Throat cancer
Gastrointestinal	Esophagus cancer Pancreatic cancer Renal carcinoma Bladder cancer Colon cancer Peptic ulcer disease
Musculoskeletal	Fractures of hip, wrist and vertebrae Osteoporosis
Gynecologic and childbirth-related	Spontaneous abortions Prematurity Low birth weight Intrauterine growth retardation Placental abruption Cervical cancer Breast
Miscellaneous	Prostate cancer Leukemia Alzheimer's disease Cataracts

C. Physical findings may include **abnormal breath sounds and signs of vascular disease.**

CLINICAL SKILLS TIP

Nicotine stains on a patient's fingers and nails and the smell of nicotine on a patient's breath will often cue the physician about a patient's tobacco use.

RULE OUT

The physician must ascertain the presence of tobacco-related comorbidities (eg, vascular disease, heart disease, pulmonary disease).

VI. Treatment:

A. Figure 19–1 and Table 19–2 summarize the **"5 A's" approach to smoking cessation** (for details relating to a patient, see the Clinical Case presented later in this chapter).

B. **Nicotine Replacement Therapy (NRT):** NRT has proved to increase the rate of success of smoking cessation; the physician should encourage patients to use it, except in special circumstances (Table 19–3).

CLINICAL CASE

A 32-year-old man presents for a pre-employment physical examination that is mandated by a prospective employer. The patient has no complaints and states that he is well. Upon further questioning, you learn that he has a frequent cough. He says that over the past few years the cough has become more productive, with about 1 teaspoon of a clear yellow-colored sputum every morning. He never has a fever and has not missed any work because of the cough. He is not overly concerned, but would like to know if there is anything that can be done about it. He has not traveled recently. He has no past medical history and takes no medications. He reluctantly tells you that he smokes 1 pack of cigarettes per day. He started smoking at age 14 and has been smoking ever since. Previously, he smoked 2 packs per day, but he has tried to cut back over the past few years. He would be happy to be a nonsmoker, but it is not clear that he is willing to quit at this time. On physical examination, his vital signs are normal and his BMI is 24. HEENT examination is non-contributory. Findings on the pulmonary examination reveal coarse upper airways sounds. There are no findings on his cardiovascular and physical examinations.

Although this patient came to see the physician for a specific purpose (pre-employment physical examination), he presents an important opportunity for the primary care physician to assess health risks. In particular, the physician can ascertain this patient's particular risks related to tobacco use. **The challenging issue for the physician is to assist this patient in quitting smoking.**

The United States Public Health Service (USPHS) has guidelines regarding tobacco cessation counseling and focuses on **5 steps, known as the "5 A's":**

1. ***Ask:*** Identify and document tobacco use status for every patient at every visit.
2. ***Advise:*** In a clear, strong, and personalized manner, urge every tobacco user to quit.
3. ***Assess:*** Is the tobacco user willing to make a quit attempt at this time?
4. ***Assist:*** For the patient willing to make a quit attempt, assist the patient in arranging counseling and in prescribing pharmacotherapy to help him/her quit.
5. ***Arrange:*** Schedule follow-up contact, in person or by telephone, preferably within the first week after the quit date.

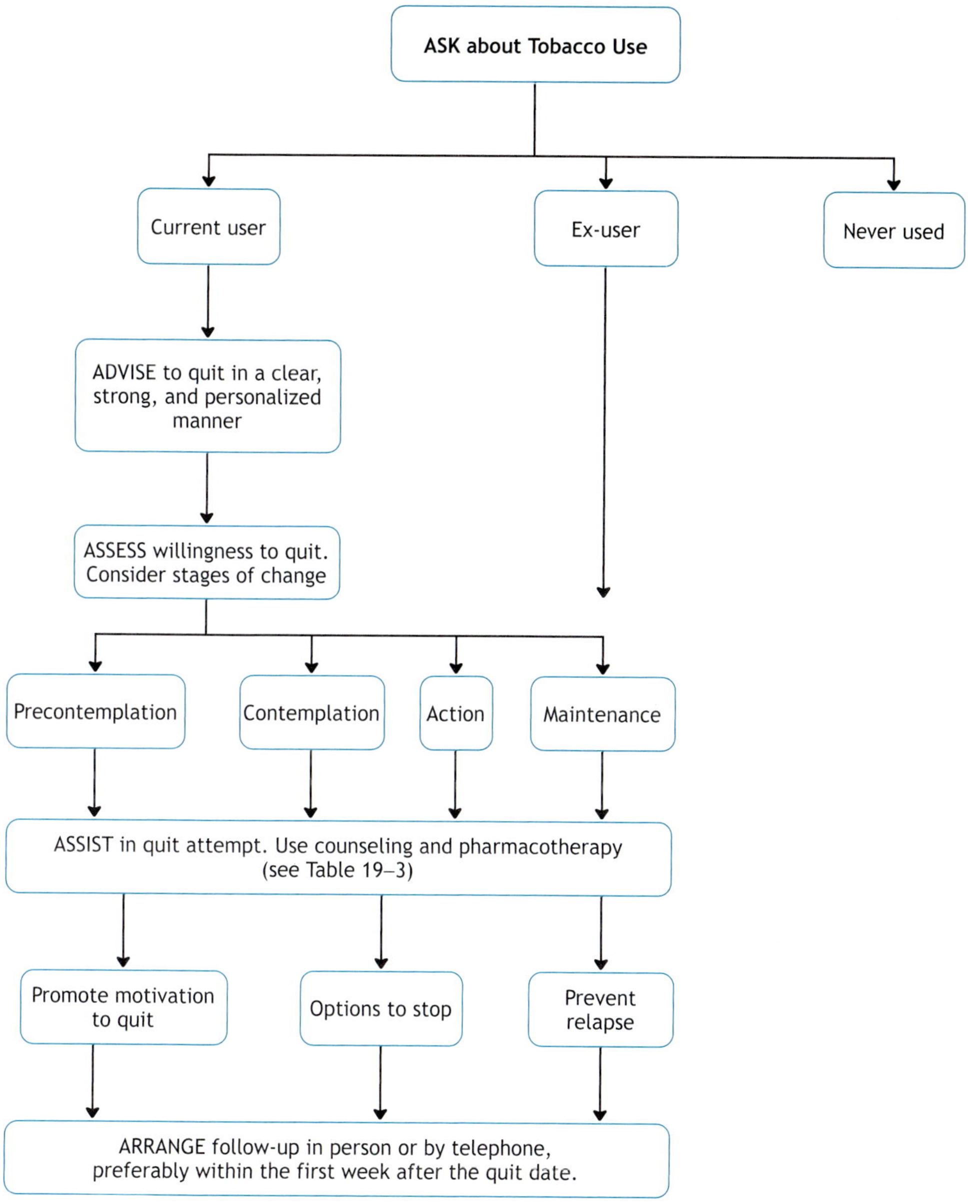

Figure 19-1. The 5 A's Approach to smoking cessation intervention.

Table 19–2. The "5 A's" approach to smoking cessation.

Ask	Identify and document tobacco use status for every patient at every visit.
Advise	In a clear, strong and personalized manner, urge every tobacco user to quit.
Assess	Is the tobacco user willing to make a quit attempt at this time?
Assist	For the patient willing to make a quit attempt, use counseling and pharmacotherapy to help him or her quit.
Arrange	Schedule follow up contact, in person or by telephone, preferably within the first week after the quit date.

Table 19–3. United States Public Health Service guidelines for Nicotine Replacement Therapy (NRT).

Who should receive pharmacotherapy for smoking cessation?	All smokers trying to quit. Special consideration should be given before using pharmacotherapy in selected populations: patients with medical contraindications; those smoking < 10 cigarettes/day; pregnant; and adolescent smokers
Which first-line pharmacotherapies are recommended in this guideline?	All 5 of the FDA-approved pharmacotherapies for smoking cessation are recommended, including bupropion SR, nicotine gum, nicotine inhaler, nicotine nasal spray, and the nicotine patch
What factors should a physician consider when choosing among the 5 first-line pharmacotherapies?	Because of the lack of sufficient data to rank-order these 5 medications, choice of a specific first-line pharmacotherapy must be guided by factors such as physician familiarity with the medications, contraindications for selected patients, patient preference, previous patient experience with a specific pharmacotherapy (positive or negative), and patient characteristics (e.g., history of depression, concerns about weight gain)
Are pharmacotherapeutic treatments appropriate for lighter smokers (eg, 10–15 cigarettes/day)?	If pharmacotherapy is use for patients who are considered "lighter smokers," physicians should consider reducing the dose of first-line pharmacotherapies
Which second-line pharmacotherapies are recommended in this guideline?	Clonidine and nortriptyline
When should second-line agents be used for treating tobacco dependence?	Consider prescribing second-line agents for patients unable to use first-line medications because of contraindications or for patients for whom first-line medications are not helpful. Monitor patients for the known side effects of second-line agents

(continued)

Table 19–3. United States Public Health Service guidelines for Nicotine Replacement Therapy (NRT). (continued)

Which pharmacotherapies should be considered for patients particularly concerned about weight gain?	Bupropion SR and NRTs, in particular nicotine gum, have been shown to delay, but not prevent, weight gain
Which pharmacotherapies should be considered for patients with a history of depression?	Bupropion SR and nortriptyline appear to be effective with this population
Should NRTs be avoided in patients with a history of cardiovascular disease?	No. NRTs are safe and have not been shown to cause adverse cardiovascular effects in patients with cardiovascular disease. However, the safety of these products has not been established for the immediate post-myocardial infarction period or in patients with severe or unstable angina
Can tobacco dependence pharmacotherapies be used long-term (eg, ≥ 6 months)?	Yes. This approach may be helpful for smokers who report persistent withdrawal symptoms during the course of pharmacotherapy or who desire long-term therapy. A minority of individuals who successfully quit smoking use ad libitum NRT medications (gum, nasal spray, and inhaler) long-term. The use of these medications long-term does not present a known health risk. Additionally, the FDA has approved the use of bupropion SR for a long-term maintenance indication
Can NRTs ever be combined?	Yes. There is evidence that combining the nicotine patch with either nicotine gum or nicotine nasal spray increases long-term abstinence rates over those produced by a single form of NRT

The smoking status of every adult should be identified and prominently documented in the medical record. For current smokers and those who have quit within the past year, smoking status should be updated at each visit. **Determine if the patient**

1. Does not smoke
2. Does smoke
3. Recently quit smoking (< 1 year)

Ask the patient, "Do you currently smoke?" If he/she says no ask, "Have you quit in the past year?" Ask adults accompanying children, "Does anyone in your/this child's household smoke?" Ask children over the age of 10, "Have you ever smoked a cigarette?" Positively reinforce nonsmoking, particularly in adolescents. Place a smoking status and/or second-hand smoke sticker on the master problem list or electronically document in computerized notes in the patient's chart. For identified smokers and recent quitters (within 1 year), update smoking status at each visit. A smoking history can be completed by people while waiting to see the physician. This assessment would gather information on addiction level, readiness to quit, prior quit attempts, and barriers to cessation. Attach the completed form to the person's chart or record for the physician/nurse review (where relevant). Regularly revise smoking status and document, including date.

Assess is extremely important. Determine the willingness of the smoker to make an attempt to quit smoking by asking him how he feels about his smoking. The purpose of determining a person's willingness to quit is to enable the most appropriate and beneficial assistance to facilitate smoking cessation. Smoking cessation is a process that occurs over time. A commonly accepted model is the **"stages of change" model** in which smokers are seen as moving through a series of stages:

1. **Precontemplative** (not considering quitting); TO
2. **Contemplative** (planning to quit within the next 6 months); TO
3. **Action** (ready to quit soon); TO
4. **Maintenance/relapse**

Ask:

1. "How do you feel about your smoking?"
2. "What do you know about the effects of smoking on health?"
3. "Have you ever thought of giving up smoking?"
4. "What would it take for you to quit?"

If the person clearly states that he/she is unwilling to make a quit attempt at this time, provide relevant information and assure them that their healthcare team is available to help when ready. For smokers not wanting to quit, remember:

1. When comparing quitting smoking with curing a disease, **physicians often do not take into account the highly addictive nature of nicotine** and the smoking habit reinforced by millions of inhalations that is strongly bound up with lifestyle habits over many years.
2. **Change** is a process that takes time; it is not an "all or nothing" phenomenon.
3. **Success** is progress through the stages, not just the act of quitting.
4. Persons in all stages of change can be helped.
5. **Intervention** must be matched to the stage of change.
6. **Relapse** is a normal part of the process, not a failure.

The next step is to advise: Provide brief cessation messages at nearly every encounter. These messages should be clear, strong, and personalized, supportive, and non-confrontational. Specifically, **advice should be**

1. **Clear:** "I think it is important for you to quit smoking and I can help you."
2. **Strong:** "As your doctor/health professional, I need you to know that quitting smoking is the most important thing you can do to protect your health now and in the future. We (the staff and I) will help you."
3. **Personalized:** Associate smoking with current health/illness, significant life events, social and economic costs, motivation level, readiness to quit, and/or the impact of second-hand smoke on children and others in the household. "I know you're concerned about your cough and that your son gets so many colds. If you stop smoking, your cough should improve and your son might get fewer colds as well."

The next step is to assist. Physicians need to provide assistance appropriate to the person's readiness to quit. Relevant information is important for everyone, even those not ready to quit. We should provide additional support for those with some interest in quitting.

If your patients are not considering quitting at this time, advise them that their health care providers are available when they are ready to quit. You can provide written materials and discuss the effects of second-hand smoke on children. If they are planning to quit but not soon, advise them that the health care team is available to help them. Encourage them to talk about the quitting process.

If they are ready to quit within the next month, do all of the above and help them **develop a quit plan.**

1. Set a quit date.
2. Tell family, friends, and coworkers about quitting and request understanding and support.
3. Anticipate challenges to planned quit attempt.
4. Remove tobacco products from the environment.

Provide practical counseling (problem-solving/skills training):

1. **Total abstinence is essential:** "You cannot have even a single puff after the quit date."
2. **Identify what helped and what hurt in previous quit attempts.**
3. **Discuss challenges/triggers** and how the patient will successfully overcome them.
4. Since alcohol can trigger relapse, the patient should **consider limiting/abstaining from alcohol** while quitting.
5. Quitting is more difficult when there is another smoker in the household. Patients should **encourage house mates to quit** with them or not smoke in their presence.
6. **Recommend pharmacotherapy,** as appropriate.
7. If a patient is a member of a special **high-risk population** (eg, adolescent or a pregnant smoker), consider providing **additional information and support.**
8. **Arrange follow-up.**

Preventing relapse can be particularly challenging. Reinforce the importance of permanent cessation at every visit. Health professionals should be aware that personal circumstances can make it difficult for people to remain as a "quitters" and inquire about these circumstances. Make people aware of major triggers, including stress and alcohol. Use open-ended questions to **identify what precipitated or is precipitating the relapse** and encourage active discussion to identify strategies to overcome these. **Problems could include**

1. Lack of support for cessation.
2. Negative mood or depression.
3. Strong or prolonged withdrawal symptoms.
4. Weight gain.
5. Flagging motivation/feeling deprived.

Encourage nicotine replacement therapy (NRT) for appropriate patients (see Table 19–3).

The final step in the 5 A's approach is to arrange appropriate follow-up for all smokers who

1. Are not considering quitting.
2. Are planning to quit but not soon.

3. Are ready to quit within the next month.
4. Have recently quit as relapse prevention or who have recently relapsed.

Arrange follow-up (in person or by phone) with smokers who are ready to quit:

1. First follow-up within the first week.
2. Second follow-up within the first month
3. To reinforce staying "quit" during visits in the first year post-cessation.

Actions to take during follow-up contact include congratulating success. If smoking has occurred, review circumstances and elicit recommitment to total abstinence. Remind the patient that a lapse can be used as a learning experience. Identify problems already encountered and anticipate challenges in the immediate future. Assess pharmacotherapy use and problems.

Review NRT, bupropion, or nortriptyline dosage and adjust if there are symptoms of overdose or inadequate dosage (see Table 19–3). People who do smoke during the first 2 weeks of cessation do not do as well as those who do not smoke during this time.

Smoking cessation is a challenge for both the physician and the patient. Physicians must include tobacco cessation in every visit and work with every patient who smokes.

CLINICAL PEARLS

Always ask the patient about smoking and use the 5 steps provided by the USPHS.

CHAPTER 20
SOMATOFORM DISORDERS

I. Defining Features (Table 20–1)

A. Somatoform disorder is a **chronic condition in which there are numerous physical complaints** caused by psychological problems for which **no underlying physical problem can be identified.** Physical complaints may last for years and result in substantial impairment.

B. The **physical symptoms** of somatoform disorders **may involve 1 or more organ systems;** physical symptoms are not intentional.

C. The patient's complaints will exceed objective findings.

D. A correlation of symptom development and psychosocial stress will be seen.

E. There is usually a **combination of biogenetic and developmental patterns.**

F. General medical conditions with multiple and confusing somatic symptoms are in the differential diagnosis.

II. Epidemiology

A. Somatoform disorders are common in primary care practice, with a prevalence of 0.2–11.6%.

B. About 26% of primary care patients meet the criteria for diagnosis of somatic "preoccupation."

C. **Onset** of a somatoform disorder is **usually before age 30.**

D. **Hypochondriasis**, a form of somatoform disorder, has a prevalence of 0.8–4.5%

III. Pathophysiology: Although the exact pathophysiology of somatoform disorders is unknown, primary somatoform disorders can be explained as follows:

A. They are associated with a **heightened awareness of normal bodily sensations.** This heightened awareness may be paired with a cognitive bias to interpret any physical symptom as indicative of medical illness.

B. **Autonomic arousal** may be heightened in some patients with somatization. This autonomic arousal may be associated with physiologic effects of endogenous noradrenergic compounds such as tachycardia or gastric hypermotility.

C. **Heightened arousal** also may induce muscle tension and pain associated with muscular hyperactivity, as seen in muscle tension headaches.

Table 20–1. Somatoform disorders.

Disorder	Symptom Presentation	Type of Symptoms	Prevalence and Gender Ratios	Voluntary Control over Symptoms	Symptom Duration	Age of Onset
Somatization disorder	Sees self as sickly; frequent medical care	Multiple systems or functions of several types, including pain and pseudo-neurologic	0.2–2% in women < 0.2% in men	No	Chronic, recurring and/or stable	Adolescence or early 20s; rare in elderly persons
Undifferentiated somatoform disorder	Sees self as ill; frequent medical care	Single system of symptom	Common	No	> 6 months	Early 20s
Conversion disorder	Onset after acute stress	Single, pseudo-neurologic	0.01–0.1; much more common in women	No	Sudden onset; short duration	Adolescence
Pain disorder	Focus solely on pain; pain behaviors	Pain; low back, neck, pelvic; emotional changes	Common	No	Sudden onset; Worsens with time	All ages; 30s–40s most common

Hypochondriasis	Fearful of disease; Preoccupied with symptoms; not reassured	Multiple; normal bodily sensations; may be vague	4–9% of medical practices; equal	No	Long history, worsens after actual illness	Any age; typically early adulthood; concerns without fears not abnormal in elderly persons
Body dysmorphic disorder	Excessive concern over imagined defect in appearance	Specific complaints of defect	?	No	Usually several years	Adolescence; early 20s
Factitious disorder with physical symptoms	Multiple operations; infections	Non-healing and unremitting	Rare	Yes	Chronic; multiple admissions; remits with confrontation	Early adulthood
Malingering	Protest; demand for medical help	Vague pain and/ or paralysis common	?	Yes	Multiple episodes of same problem	Early adulthood

D. To some degree, somatoform symptoms are normal; bodily experiences of emotions are common.

IV. Classification of Somatoform Disorders

A. **Somatization disorder** is characterized by **multiple physical complaints referable to several organ systems.** Anxiety, panic disorder, and depression are often present. Major depression is an important consideration in the differential diagnosis.

1. History begins **before age 30,** occurs over a period of several years, and results in treatment being sought.
2. There is significant **impairment in social, occupational, or other important areas of functioning.**
3. Each of the following criteria must have been met, with individual symptoms occurring at any time during the course of the disturbance.
   a. **Four pain symptoms:** A history of pain related to at least 4 sites or functions (eg, head, abdomen, back, joints, extremities, chest, rectum, during sexual intercourse, during menstruation, or during urination).
   b. **Two gastrointestinal symptoms:** A history of at least 2 gastrointestinal symptoms other than pain (eg, nausea, diarrhea, bloating, vomiting other than during pregnancy, or intolerance of several different foods).
   c. **One sexual symptom:** A history of at least 1 sexual or reproductive symptom other than pain (eg, sexual indifference, erectile or ejaculatory dysfunction, irregular menses, excessive menstrual bleeding, vomiting throughout pregnancy).
   d. **One pseudoneurologic symptom:** A history of at least 1 symptom or deficit suggesting a neurologic disorder not limited to pain (conversion symptoms such as blindness, double vision, deafness, loss of touch or pain sensation, hallucinations, aphonia, impaired coordination or balance, paralysis or localized weakness, difficulty swallowing, difficulty breathing, urinary retention, seizures; dissociative symptoms such as amnesia; or loss of consciousness other than fainting).

B. **Undifferentiated somatoform disorder** is for clinically significant somatoform complaints persisting > 6 months.

C. **Conversion disorder** is when the psychological conflict converts to physical symptoms in parts of the body innervated by the sensorimotor system (eg, paralysis, aphonia).

1. One or more symptoms or deficits affecting voluntary motor or sensory function suggest a **neurologic or general medical condition.**
2. **Psychological factors** are judged to be associated with the symptom or deficit because the initiation or exacerbation of the symptom or deficit is preceded by conflicts or other stressors.
3. The symptom or deficit is **not intentionally produced or feigned** (ie, factitious disorder or malingering).
4. The **symptom or deficit cannot,** after appropriate investigation, **be fully explained** by a general medical condition, or by the direct effects of a substance, or as a culturally sanctioned behavior or experience.
5. The symptom or deficit causes **clinically significant distress or impairment** in social, occupational, or other important areas of functioning or warrants medical evaluation.

6. The symptom or deficit is **not limited to pain or sexual dysfunction,** does not occur exclusively during the course of somatization disorder, and is not better accounted for by another disorder.

D. **Pain disorder associated with psychological factors** is when the patient has a long history of complaints of severe pain that is not consistent with anatomic and clinical signs.
   1. **Pain in one or more anatomical sites** is the predominant focus of the clinical presentation and is of sufficient severity to warrant clinical attention.
   2. The pain causes clinically significant **distress or impairment** in social, occupational, or other important areas of functioning.
   3. **Psychological factors** are judged to have an important role in the onset, severity, exacerbation, or maintenance of the pain.
   4. The symptom or deficit is **not intentionally produced or feigned** (as in factitious disorder or malingering).
   5. The pain is not better accounted for by a mood, anxiety, or psychotic disorder and **does not meet criteria for dyspareunia.**
   6. **Acute pain is $<$ 6 months and chronic pain is $\geq$ 6 months.**

E. **Hypochondriasis** is the fear of disease and a preoccupation with the body, with perceptual amplification and heightened responsiveness.
   1. **Preoccupation with fears of having, or ideas that a person has, a serious disease** based on the person's misinterpretations of bodily symptoms.
   2. The preoccupation persists despite appropriate medical evaluation and reassurance.
   3. The belief (criterion 1) is **not of delusional intensity** and is not restricted to a circumscribed concern about body appearance.
   4. The preoccupation causes clinically significant **distress or impairment** in social, occupational, or other important areas of functioning.
   5. The duration of the disturbance is **at least 6 months.**

F. **Body dysmorphic disorder** involves excessive preoccupation with a minor or imagined defect of 1 or more body parts.
   1. Preoccupation with an **imagined defect in appearance.** If a slight physical anomaly is present, the person's concern is markedly excessive.
   2. The preoccupation causes significant **distress or impairment** in social, occupational, or other important areas of functioning.
   3. The preoccupation is not better accounted for by another mental disorder (eg, dissatisfaction with body shape and size in anorexia nervosa).

G. **Factitious disorders** are when patients have **self-induced symptoms to try to deceive physicians.** These deceptions include self-mutilation, fever, hemorrhage, hypoglycemia, and seizures. **Münchhausen by proxy** is when a parent, most commonly a mother, creates an illness in their children.

H. **Malingering** is not a somatoform disorder per se because symptoms are voluntary and deceptive.

V. Risk Factors

A. **Genetic** factors appear to play a role in developing somatic sensitivities.

B. **Traumatic experiences** are predictive of somatoform disorders.

C. **Family history** is important since families differ in how they respond to symptoms and illnesses.

D. **Social factors** such as single parenting, living alone, unemployment, and marital and job difficulties also play a role.

VI. Clinical Presentation

A. **Symptoms of Somatoform Disorder**
  1. **Unexplained symptoms that are chronic or constantly changing**
  2. **Multiple symptoms:** 4 in males and 6 in females (eg, fainting, menstrual disturbances, headache, chest pain, dizziness, and palpitations)
  3. **Vague idiosyncratic complaints**
  4. Paradoxical **worsening of symptoms with treatment**

B. **Signs of Somatoform Disorder** (often unexplained)
  1. **Paralysis**
  2. **Signs of self-mutilation**
  3. Presence of symptoms listed above for which there are no physical examination findings.

VII. Differential Diagnosis

A. Hyperparathyroidism

B. Porphyria

C. Multiple sclerosis

D. Systemic lupus erythematosus

E. Primary or secondary depression

F. Other mental disorders, including anxiety and substance-abuse disorders

VIII. Diagnostic Findings (Figure 20–1)

A. Screening questionnaires related to **depression** should be used as well as questions about **cognitive symptoms** such as guilt.

B. Diagnosis requires a finding that the **symptoms have brought unneeded medical treatment** or that there is impairment in social, occupational, or other important areas of functioning.

C. Imaging studies are only useful to rule out unexplained physical symptoms due to a medical disorder.

D. Invasive diagnostic procedures and aggressive surgical assessments should be avoided, unless used to rule out unexplained physical symptoms due to a medical disorder.

IX. Treatment

A. **Medical**
  1. **A therapeutic physician-patient relationship should be developed.** Regular, brief appointments may be helpful. Have the patient come to the office and do not prescribe drugs (that are often abused) over the phone. It may be useful for the patient to keep a thorough diary.
  2. Somatoform disorder should be **treated as a chronic illness, with a focus on functioning rather than symptom cure.**

B. **Psychological**
  1. When the patient seems ready to undergo lifestyle changes, **small group therapy sessions with others with the same condition may be helpful.**

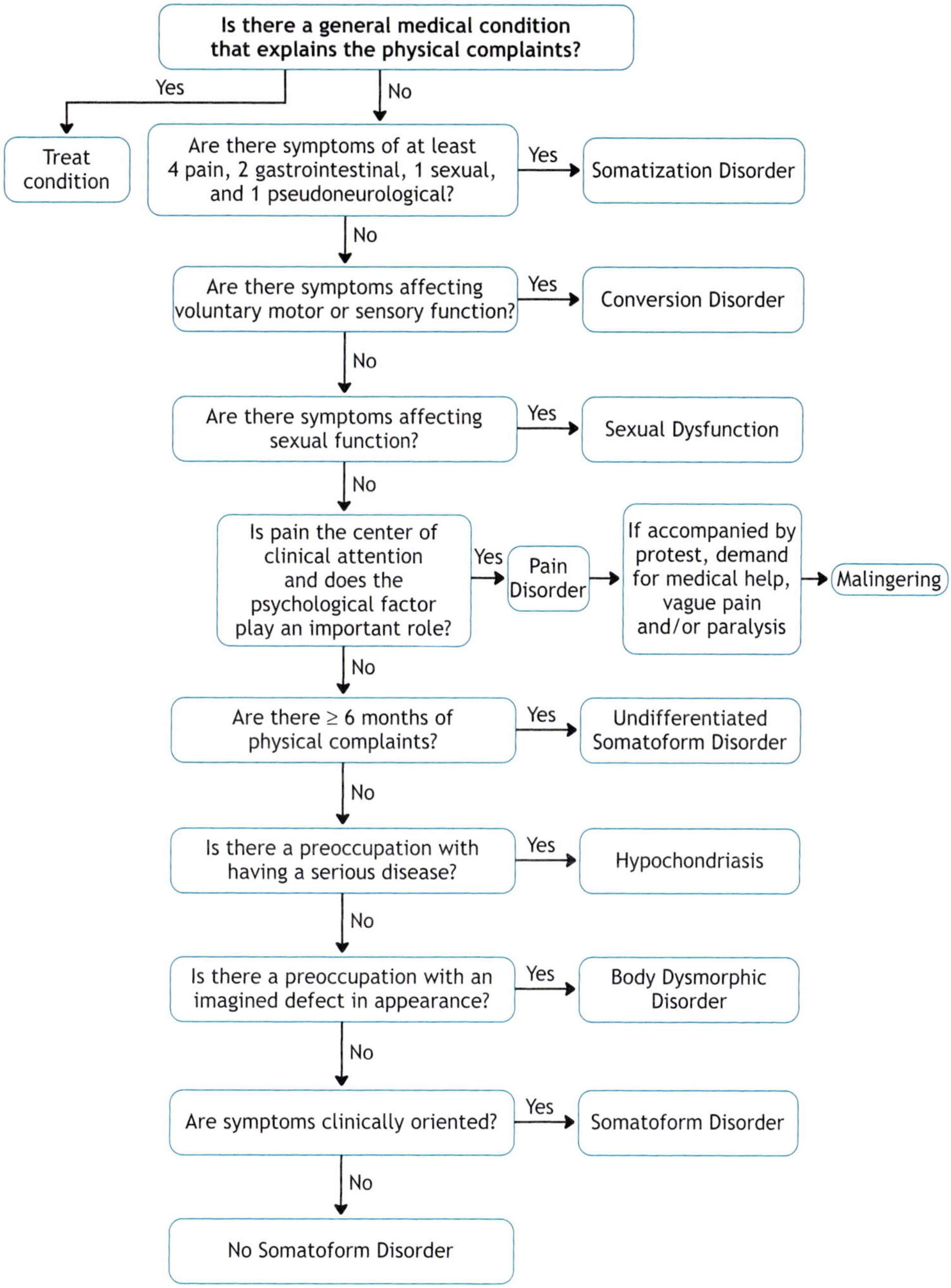

Figure 20–1. Diagnosing somatoform disorders.

2. For patients with factitious disorder, **early psychiatric treatment** is recommended. Often this disorder is a patient's cry for help, and psychiatric treatment is helpful.
3. **Cognitive behavioral therapy** is helpful in nearly 70% of patients.

C. **Behavioral**

1. This type of therapy is best exemplified by **biofeedback** techniques.
2. Patients may also benefit from **mind-body interventions**, such as massage, movement therapies, relaxation, and guided imagery.

D. **Social**

1. Social endeavors include **family, work, and other interpersonal activities.** It is helpful for family members to accompany the patient to appointments to learn how best to coexist with the patient.
2. Patients often find **peer support groups** helpful because these groups can provide a climate of encouragement and acceptance.

CLINICAL CASE

The patient is a 35-year-old woman presenting for evaluation of multiple problems. She is most concerned today about a headache. She states that the headache begins at the back of her neck and moves up to envelope her entire head in pain. There is a squeezing sensation at the temples. She rates the pain as a 5 on a scale of 1 –10. She says that the pain does not radiate, but her entire head hurts. She has tried acetaminophen and ibuprofen, but they offer no relief. She expresses significant concern that she has had these headaches for many years and no one has been able to determine a diagnosis. She tells you that she has had CT scans of her head, multiple blood tests, and a lumbar puncture, and all studies have been normal. On further questioning, she says that the headaches began when she was in her early 20s. She has also experienced intermittent abdominal pain, back pain, and occasional rectal pain with defecation. She has frequent bloating and claims intolerance to many foods. Additionally, you learn that she has lost interest in sexual relations with her husband. She tells you that she loves him very much, but feels so troubled by her ongoing problems that she has no interest in sex. She tells you that 7 years ago she experienced double vision. At the time, her physician was worried about multiple sclerosis and performed an MRI of her head. The results of the MRI were normal. She has seen many physicians, none of whom have been able to arrive at a diagnosis. Various medications have been tried as well as changes in her diet. She thinks nothing has helped, and she is now worse. Her husband is also upset, because he feels that his wife no longer enjoys socializing with their friends. She is hopeful that you will be able to find out what is wrong with her and provide her with appropriate therapy. On physical examination, her vital signs are normal. She appears in no acute distress. Her heart, lungs, and abdomen are all normal. A neurologic examination is also normal. Her affect seems appropriate as does her mental status.

Patients presenting to a primary care physician's office with undifferentiated symptoms can be difficult to diagnose. However, as challenging as it may be, primary care physicians are in the best position to appropriately care for these patients. Care must include continuity of care and attention to the physician-patient relationship (see IX and Table 20–1).

This patient's problems are related to a somatoform disorder. Somatoform symptoms exist on a continuum and should not be explained solely as a mental disorder.

The physician should take a **detailed history of the patient,** which will demonstrate the importance of the physician-patient relationship. Similarly, the physical examination should be detailed and particularly the neurologic examination. Laboratory investigations should be limited. If indicated, **specific studies used to rule out somatization due to general medical conditions** can include the following:

1. **Thyroid-stimulating hormone (TSH)**
2. **Urine drug screen,** including cannabis, amphetamine, hallucinogens, cocaine, opioids, and benzodiazepines
3. **Blood studies:** Screen for occult alcoholism.
4. **Psychological testing:** Minnesota Multiphasic Personality Inventory (MMPI) may provide insight into the likelihood of a somatoform disorder. Negative MMPI studies should encourage further pursuit of a medical cause for the symptoms.

CLINICAL SKILLS TIP

Patients who ultimately are found to have a somatoform disorder are the most challenging to physicians because their presenting complaint is often associated with serious biomedical disease such as chest pain.

CHAPTER 21

URINARY TRACT INFECTIONS

I. Defining Features

A. A single pathogen is found in acute urinary tract infections (UTIs), and 2 or more pathogens are found in chronic cases.

B. **Coliform bacteria** are responsible for most non-nosocomial, uncomplicated UTIs.

C. ***Escherichia coli*** is the most common form of coliform bacteria found in UTIs.

II. Epidemiology

A. Urinary tract infections are **more common in women.**

B. About 50% of women have at least 1 UTI in their lifetime.

C. About 3–8% of women have bacteriuria at any given time in the urinary tract.

D. **About 25% of women with a simple UTI experience recurrence of the infection within 6 months.**

E. UTIs account for 7 million physician visits a year.

F. UTIs are uncommon in men younger than age 50 years. There are 8 infections per 10,000 men aged 21–50 years.

G. Bacteriuria develops in 10–15% of hospitalized patients with **indwelling urethral catheters,** and the risk of UTIs is about 3–5% per day of catheterization.

H. UTIs are the most common cause of infection in **nursing home residents.**

I. With more **frequent sexual activity** enteric or coliform bacteria will enter the woman's short urethra during intercourse.

III. Pathophysiology

A. **Ascending infection with enteric flora** is common in women because of urethral colonization with fecal and vaginal flora and the short urethra.

B. **Inflammation of the bladder wall and trigone** causes urinary frequency, urgency, dysuria, and a sensation of incomplete emptying.

C. Infection in men suggests an anatomic, usually **obstructing abnormality.**

D. If bacteria ascend from the bladder, infection involving the renal medulla and collecting system develops and is called **pyelonephritis.**

IV. Risk Factors

A. Women

1. Previous UTIs
2. Diabetes mellitus
3. Pregnancy
4. Poor anal hygiene or back to front wiping
5. More frequent or vigorous sexual activity than usual or use of spermicides or diaphragm
6. Underlying abnormalities of the urinary tract (eg, tumor, calculi, stricture, incomplete bladder emptying, or presence of bladder posterior valve abnormalities)

B. Men

1. Benign prostatic hypertrophy (BPH)
2. Urinary or fecal incontinence
3. Recent urologic surgery
4. Catheterization or instrumentation
5. Outlet obstruction
6. Immunocompromised host

V. Clinical Presentation

A. Signs and Symptoms of UTIs in Women

1. Dysuria or pain during urination
2. Urgency and frequency
3. Sensation of incomplete bladder emptying
4. Hematuria
5. Lower abdominal pain or cramping
6. Offensive odor of urine
7. Nocturia

B. Signs and Symptoms of UTIs in Men

1. Dysuria or pain during urination
2. Urgency and frequency
3. Hesitancy
4. Slow urinary stream
5. Dribbling of urine
6. Nocturia
7. Suprapubic discomfort
8. Low back pain
9. Hematuria
10. Systemic symptoms (eg, chills, fever) with concomitant pyelonephritis or prostatitis

CLINICAL SKILLS TIP

Although frequency, urgency, and dysuria are common symptoms of uncomplicated UTIs, be wary of patients who report fever and flank or low back pain because these signs and symptoms point to pyelonephritis.

VI. Differential Diagnosis

A. Women

1. **Vulvovaginitis:** Distinguish by pelvic examination and urinalysis
2. **Pelvic inflammatory disease** (PID): Distinguish by pelvic examination and urinalysis
3. **Sexually transmitted disease** (STD) causing urethritis or pyuria
4. **Hematuria** from causes other than infection (eg, neoplasia, calculi)
5. **Interstitial cystitis**
6. Psychological dysfunction

B. Men

1. **Urethritis and prostatitis** (urethral discharge or prostatic tenderness): Distinguish by physical examination
2. **Anatomic or functional pathology**
3. Infections in other sites of the genitourinary tract (eg, epididymis)

RULE OUT

Although a patient with an uncomplicated UTI may have hematuria, its presence demands a complete investigation of the genitourinary tract, including imaging and cystoscopy of the upper part of the tract to determine if there is a tumor.

VII. Diagnostic Findings

A. Laboratory Studies

1. **Women**
   a. **Urinalysis demonstrating pyuria** (> 10 neutrophils per high power field on microscopic examination): **Leukocyte esterase dipsticks** are useful but fail to detect pyuria in up to 20% of patients. False-positives occur when vaginal leukocytes are present.
   b. **Urinalysis demonstrating bacteriuria** (any amount on unspun urine, or 10 rod-shaped bacteria per high power field on centrifuged urine): **Nitrite dipsticks** are useful (and 94% specific), but fail to detect bacteriuria in 30–50% of patients. Nitrite dipsticks may be negative in patients who do not eat meat.
   c. **Urine culture demonstrating growth of single species of bacteria:** Suspect contaminated specimen when culture shows multiple types of bacteria.
   d. **Urine culture to rule out infection:** If a dipstick test is negative in patients with atypical symptoms, culture should still be performed.
2. **Men**
   a. **Urinalysis demonstrating pyuria** (> 10 neutrophils per high power field on microscopic exam). **Leukocyte esterase dipsticks** are useful but fail to detect pyuria in up to 20% of patients.
   b. **Urinalysis demonstrating bacteriuria** (any amount on unspun urine, or 10 rod-shaped bacteria per high power field on centrifuged urine): **Nitrite dipsticks** are useful (and 94% specific), but fail to detect bacteriuria in 30–50% of patients. Nitrite dipsticks may be negative in patients who do not eat meat.
   c. **Urine dipstick leukocyte esterase** (75–90% sensitivity, 95% specificity), and nitrate (35–85% sensitivity, 70% specificity).

d. **Urine culture:** 10 per high power colonies of pathogens (or counts > 100,000 bacteria/mL of urine) confirms diagnosis (eg, *E coli, Klebsiella, Pseudomonas*). **Lower counts can be indicative of infection, especially if pyuria is present.**

B. **Imaging Studies**

1. **Women and Men**
   a. Ultrasound
   b. Cystoscopy
   c. Intravenous pyelography
2. **Infants, Children, and Older Patients with Recurrent Infections**
   a. **Ultrasound** imaging is the first test of choice.
   b. For infants and children, obtain ultrasound and if ureteral dilation detected, obtain either **voiding cystourethrogram** or **isotope cystogram** to detect reflux.

C. **Diagnostic Procedures**

1. **Suprapubic bladder aspiration or urethral catheterization** to obtain urine specimen from infants and neonates.
2. **Urethral catheterization** to obtain urine specimen from children and adults if voided urine is suspected of being contaminated.
3. **No urine culture** is needed for diagnosis of non-pregnant young adult women with first episode of UTI and classic symptoms. Obtain **urinalysis and culture** in other age groups, if repeat episode, if pregnant, or if symptoms are not classic.

VIII. Treatment (Figure 21–1)

A. **Common Treatment Modalities for Women and Men**

1. Maintain good hydration and prescribe analgesic, if required.
2. Discontinue sexual activity until symptom-free.
3. Patient with indwelling catheter
   a. If symptomatic (fever, sepsis, or other systemic symptoms) of **acute infection, institute treatment.** If the patient **resides in an institution** and the institution has > 20% *E coli* resistance to trimethoprim-sulfamethoxazole, consider choosing an alternate first-line treatment such as
      (1) Nitrofurantoin
      (2) Ciprofloxacin
   b. Patients who have chronic indwelling urinary catheters **always have colonization of urine,** usually with multiple bacterial species. If **asymptomatic bacterial colonization,** there is **no need to treat** (sterilization of urine not possible and resistant organisms can take up residence).

B. **Specific Treatment Considerations for Women**

1. For the patient with an **uncomplicated UTI,** most protocols recommend a **short (3–5 days) course of antibiotics.** First-line antibiotics include
   a. **Trimethoprim-sulfamethoxazole DS** 1 pill twice a day for 3 days
   b. **Trimethoprim** 100 mg 1 twice a day for 3 days
   c. **If allergic to sulfa or trimethoprim**, give
      (1) Nitrofurantoin (Macrobid) 100 mg twice a day for 7 days
      (2) Ciprofloxacin 250 mg twice a day for 3 days

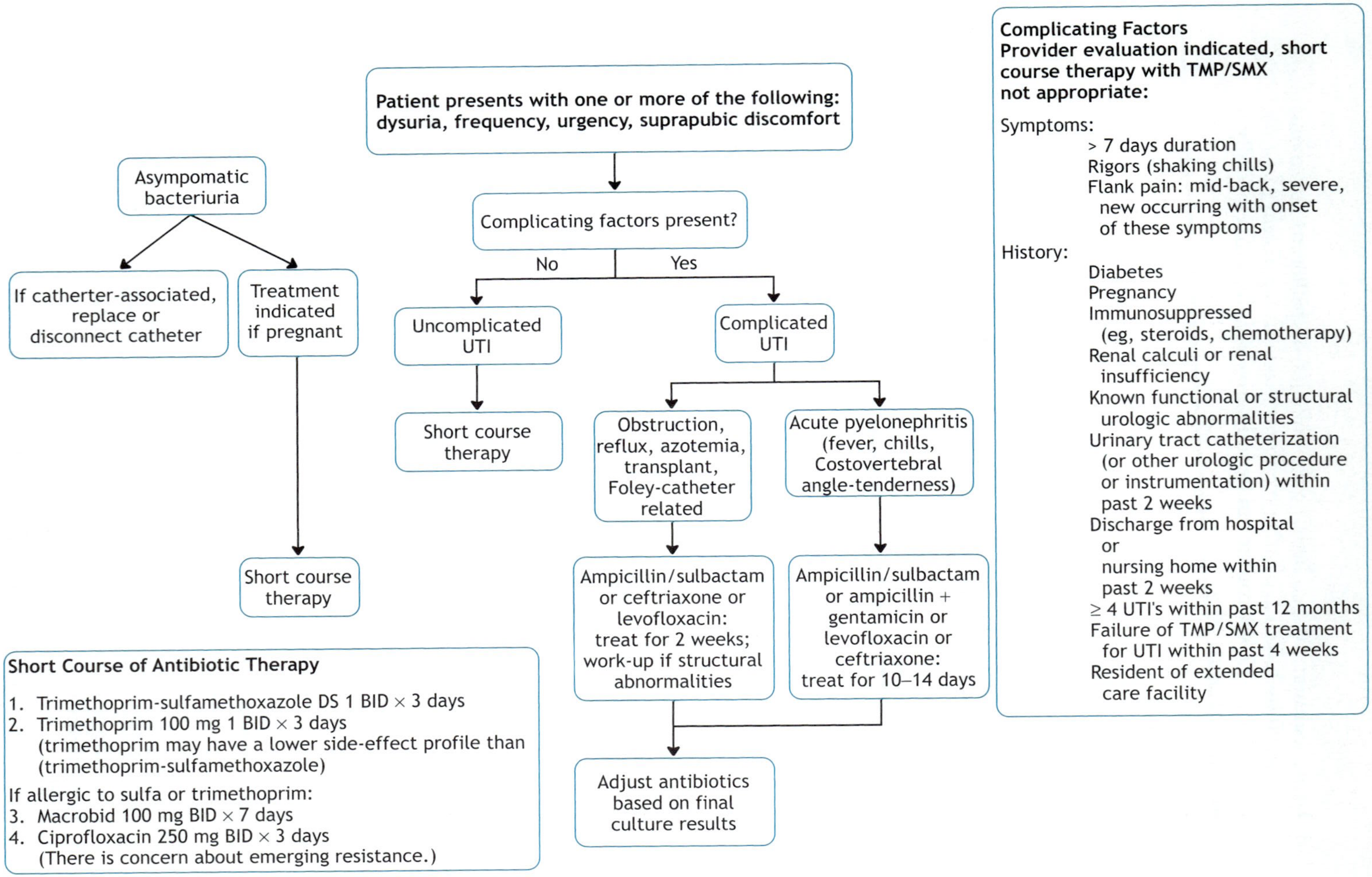

Figure 21–1. Care of the patient with symptoms of a urinary tract infection.

2. Sulfa and ciprofloxacin may cause an increase in international normalized ratio (INR) values in patients taking warfarin.
3. Women who have **recurrent UTIs** and no underlying urinary tract abnormality can be treated with **continuous low-dose antibiotic prophylaxis or postcoital prophylaxis for 3–6 months.** Trimethoprim-sulfamethoxazole, nitrofurantoin, cephalexin, or trimethoprim are effective agents.
4. **Cranberry juice** may help prevent and may treat UTIs by inhibiting bacterial adherence to bladder epithelium.

IX. Summary Table

Disease	Pathophysiology	Diagnostic Studies	Treatment
Urinary tract infection	Infectious: coliform bacteria	Urinalysis	Antibiotics
Vulvovaginitis	Infectious: fungal, bacteria, parasites	KOH or saline prep of vaginal discharge	Antibiotics
Pelvic inflammatory disease	Infectious: sexually transmitted bacteria	Pelvic exam and cultures	Antibiotics
Prostatitis	Infectious or inflammatory	Prostate exam	Antibiotics and/or anti-inflammatory agents
Epididymitis	Infectious or inflammatory	Genitourinary exam	Antibiotics

CLINICAL CASE

A 27-year-old sexually active woman presents with complaints of urinary burning and frequency. She is in a stable, mutually monogamous heterosexual relationship and uses oral contraceptive pills. She does not use alcohol or tobacco. Her past history is otherwise unremarkable. Physical examination reveals her to be non-toxic with normal vital signs. She has no costovertebral angle (CVA) tenderness.

This patient presents with very straightforward and uncomplicated symptoms suggestive of a UTI. This is certainly the most common presentation of an uncomplicated UTI. However, we must always consider less common presentations, which could include any of the following:

1. An **infant** may only present with a non-focal history and physical except for an **elevated temperature.**
2. A **pregnant patient** may present only with **frequency,** which could be thought due to the reduced bladder size associated with pregnancy.

3. Some **young women** could experience **hematuria and foul-smelling urine.**
4. Although UTIs are less common in **men,** they could present with some of the same UTI symptoms as women, as well as **dribbling of the urine and hesitancy.**
5. **Complicated UTIs** are present in patients with **comorbid conditions, indwelling Foley catheters,** and in **hospitalized or institutionalized patients.**
6. **Fever, back pain, and signs of sepsis** could also complicate the presentation, leading the physician to consider **pyelonephritis and urosepsis.**

Although this patient's physical examination was relatively complete, some protocols suggest empiric treatment without such a thorough physical examination. A young, sexually active non-pregnant woman with no comorbid conditions can generally be treated this way. Diagnostic work-up can include a dipstick urinalysis, a microscopic urinalysis, and/or a urine culture, or nothing. There are multiple sets of guidelines, but there is no consensus regarding the work-up of patients with an uncomplicated UTI. See VIII B and Figure 21–1 for a summary of treatment options.

Although short course therapy is ideal for many patients, it is important to remember the criteria for whom short course therapy would not be appropriate. Symptoms suggestive of pyelonephritis or severe infection such as long duration, rigors, flank pain, or temperature > 38.3 °C (101 °F) would make short-course therapy inappropriate. Certain medical history of the patient such as diabetes, pregnancy, immunosuppression, underlying urinary tract disease, or renal calculi, recent medical intervention (hospitalization or catheterization), or recurrent UTIs would also make short-course inappropriate. Residents of an extended-care facility should not receive short-course therapy.

CLINICAL PEARLS

Burning, urgency, and frequency are the classic symptoms in a patient with a urinary tract infection.

CHAPTER 22
VAGINITIS

I. Defining Features

A. Vaginal irritation

B. Pruritus

C. Pain

D. Unusual discharge

II. Epidemiology

A. In unselected populations, the incidence of vaginitis is as low as 4% of cases; **in clinics that treat sexually transmitted disease (STDs), the incidence of vaginitis is as high as 33% of cases.**

B. Approximately 6.5% of women older than 18 years have had at least 1 episode of candidal vaginitis during a 2-month period in 1 calendar year.

C. **African-American women are 3 times more likely to have yeast infections than are white women.**

III. Pathophysiology

A. The **normal vaginal discharge** is clear to slightly white and contains mucous, epithelial cells, and bacteria (particularly lactobacilli) and **has a pH of 4.0.**

B. A **shift from a healthy lactobacilli-based endogenous flora to an anaerobically based endogenous** flora results in an infection and/or inflammation, causing increased mucous production and exudation of white blood cells from the mucosa-producing vaginal discharge.

C. **Common Causes of Vaginitis**

1. **Bacterial vaginosis** is a clinical syndrome resulting from replacement of the normal hydrogen peroxide (H_2O_2)-producing *Lactobacillus* sp in the vagina with high concentrations of anaerobic bacteria (eg, *Prevotella* sp and *Mobiluncus* sp), *Gardnerella vaginalis,* and *Mycoplasma hominis.*
2. **Candidal vulvovaginitis** is commonly caused by *Candida albicans,* although it can also be caused by other *Candida* sp and other yeasts.
3. **Trichomoniasis** is caused by the protozoan *Trichomonas vaginalis.*
4. **Estrogen-related vulvovaginitis** is also called atrophic vaginitis and is found in the estrogen-deficient state of menopause.

5. **Prepubescent vulvovaginitis** is also related to estrogen deficiency and to poor hygiene.

D. A **rectal reservoir of organisms can result in autoinfection.**

IV. Risk Factors

A. Bacterial Vaginosis

1. Whether having multiple sexual partners is a risk factor for bacterial vaginosis remains controversial. Having a "new" sex partner or multiple sex partners can upset the normal balance of bacteria in the vagina and put women at increased risk. Treatment of the male sex partner has not been beneficial in preventing the recurrence of bacterial vaginosis.
2. Although having multiple sexual partners is controversial as a risk factor, women who have never been sexually active are rarely affected.

B. Candidal Vulvovaginitis

1. Antibiotic therapy
2. Diabetes mellitus
3. Pregnancy
4. Corticosteroid therapy
5. HIV infection
6. Occlusive synthetic underwear
7. Oral contraceptive pills (OCPs) (low dose OCPs usually do not cause increased risk of infection)
8. Hypothyroidism

C. Trichomoniasis

1. Penis-to-vagina intercourse with infected partner
2. Vulva-to-vulva contact with infected partner

D. Estrogen-related Vulvovaginitis

1. Estrogen-deficient states accompanying metabolic disorders
2. Vaginal infections caused by bacteria and fungi

E. Prepubescent Vulvovaginitis

1. Co-existing pharyngitis or other systemic conditions
2. Faulty hygiene
3. Trauma

V. Clinical Presentation

A. Signs and Symptoms of Bacterial Vaginosis

1. Thin gray-white vaginal discharge, mildly adherent to vaginal walls
2. Vaginal discharge demonstrating pH > 4.5 and clue cells in wet mount
3. Musty or fishy smelling vaginal discharge, exacerbated by intercourse
4. Vaginal and/or vulvar irritation
5. Frothy discharge

B. Signs and Symptoms of Candidal Vulvovaginitis

1. Thick curd-like vaginal discharge
2. Erythema of vulva
3. Thick white patches attached to vaginal mucosa
4. Inflamed vulvar tissue
5. Intense vulvar itching

6. Erythema, pain, and pruritus of crural and perineal area
7. Dyspareunia

C. Signs and Symptoms of Trichomoniasis

1. Vulvar irritation
2. Punctate hemorrhages on the vagina and cervix
3. Diffuse, malodorous, yellow-green discharge
4. Burning and itching
5. Dyspareunia

D. Signs and Symptoms of Estrogen-related Vulvovaginitis

1. Vulvar thinning of epidermis and decreased integrity of supporting structures; thinning and atrophy often produces pruritus.
2. Vaginal dryness
3. Decreased vaginal secretions
4. Dyspareunia

E. Signs and Symptoms of Prepubescent Vulvovaginitis

1. Irritation and erythema of vulva
2. Vaginal discharge
3. Excoriation
4. Bleeding
5. Offensive odor
6. Itching

CLINICAL SKILLS TIP

Be certain to ask the patient if she has already tried an over-the-counter treatment for candidal vaginitis. If she has, you should consider a diagnosis of a different cause of the vaginitis.

VI. Differential Diagnosis

A. Bacterial Vulvovaginitis

1. Gonorrhea (*Neisseria gonorrhoeae*)
2. Chlamydial infection (*Chlamydia trachomatis*)
3. *Escherichia coli* vaginitis
4. Staphylococci vaginitis
5. Fungal vaginitis
6. Atrophic vaginitis

B. Candidal Vulvovaginitis

1. Gonorrheal vaginitis (in prepubertal girls)
2. Pinworm vaginitis
3. Contact dermatitis/vaginitis
4. Complicated vulvovaginal candidiasis (VVC)

C. Estrogen-related Vulvovaginitis

1. Neoplasia
2. Vulvar dystrophies

D. Prepubescent Vulvovaginitis

1. Contact dermatitis
2. Eczema
3. Psoriasis

RULE OUT

Patients who have vaginal neoplasms may present with vaginal discharge. A neoplasm would show a mass in the vagina and may be primary or secondary to carcinoma of the uterus, rectum, bladder, or external genitalia.

VII. Diagnostic Findings

A. Laboratory Studies

1. **Bacterial Vaginosis**
   a. **pH paper:** pH is > 4.5.
   b. **Wet prep:** Clue cells in > 10–20% of epithelial cells and fewer white blood cells than epithelial cells.
   c. **10% KOH solution:** Applying KOH to the slide of secretions will demonstrate a transient amine or fishy odor ("Whiff test").
   d. **Gram stain** indicates absence of lactobacilli.
2. **Candidal Vulvovaginitis**
   a. **10% KOH solution:** Yeast, spores, and/or pseudohyphae are seen on smear.
   b. **Culture findings on Nickerson's or Sabouraud's media:** usually only indicated for recurrent infections.
   c. **pH paper:** Vaginal pH is < 4.5.
3. **Trichomoniasis**
   a. **Saline prep:** Shows flagellated ovoid protozoa
   b. **pH:** > 5.0
4. **Estrogen-related Vulvovaginitis**
   a. **Cytology for maturation index:** Low maturation index signifying a decreased turnover of cells from decreased estrogen effect.
   b. **Follicle-stimulating hormone (FSH):** Elevated in perimenopausal or menopausal women.
   c. **Estradiol level:** Decreased in perimenopausal or menopausal women.
5. **Prepubescent Vulvovaginitis**
   a. **Cervical culture** for bacteria or viruses
   b. **Vaginal culture** for fungi
   c. **Gram stain** of cervical secretion
   d. **Rectal tape examination** for pinworms
   e. **Potassium hydroxide and saline smears** for fungi, clue cells and trichomonads

B. Diagnostic Procedures

1. **Bacterial Vaginosis** (none)
2. **Candidal Vulvovaginitis**
   a. **Smear of discharge with 10% KOH solution:** hyphae
   b. **Pap smear**
3. **Trichomoniasis**
   a. **Saline prep of vaginal discharge**
   b. **Pap smear** (although saline prep must be used as confirmatory)
4. **Estrogen-related Vulvovaginitis**
   a. **Examination of vagina and vulva:** maturation index
   b. **FSH level:** Confirm menopause
   c. **Estradiol level:** Evaluate circulating estrogen level

5. **Prepubescent Vulvovaginitis**
   a. Place child in knee-chest position for best result. Hold buttocks apart and slightly upward.
   b. Visualization of the vagina may be necessary using a nasal speculum or infant laryngoscope.
   c. If blood or foul-smelling discharge is present, visualization is mandatory.

VIII. Treatment (Figure 22–1)

A. Bacterial Vaginosis: Pharmacotherapy

1. Metronidazole (Flagyl)
2. Metronidazole vaginal gel
3. Clindamycin

B. Candidal Vulvovaginitis

1. Remove foreign body, if present.
2. Recommend povidone-iodine (Betadine, Operand) douche 12–30 mL/L of water daily for symptomatic relief until specific therapy is effective.
3. **If urination causes burning,** have patient
   a. Urinate through a tubular device such as a toilet-paper roll or a plastic cup with the end cut out.
   b. Pour warm water over vaginal area while urinating.
4. If the patient is diabetic, strict control of blood glucose is necessary.
5. If patient has recurrent infections, limit sweets (sucrose) and dairy products (lactose).
6. Avoid overexertion and heat and excessive sweating.
7. Abstain from sexual relations until therapy has been completed and patient is asymptomatic.
8. **Pharmacotherapy**
   a. Fluconazole
   b. Miconazole nitrate (Monistat)
   c. Butoconazole nitrate (Femstat)
   d. Terconazole (Terazol)
   e. Clotrimazole (Gyne-Lotrimin)

C. Trichomoniasis

1. Abstain from sex until patient and partner are treated and asymptomatic.
2. **Pharmacotherapy for both patient and partner:** Treating both patient and her partner with either of the following drugs will result in a cure rate of 90–95%.
   a. Metronidazole 2 gm orally in a single dose
   b. Metronidazole 500 mg twice a day for 7 days

D. Estrogen-related Vulvovaginitis

1. **Estrogen replacement therapy (ERT)** will lessen and reverse symptoms and aid in reversing the thinning of the squamous epithelial layer. ERT results in increased blood supply to the genital tissues.
2. Symptomatic relief, if needed (eg, cool baths or compresses)
3. A variety of **estrogen preparations** are available.
   a. Estrogen conjugated (Premarin) 0.625 mg daily
   b. Estradiol (Estrace) 1 mg daily
   c. Estradiol (Estraderm) patch 0.05 mg, changed twice weekly

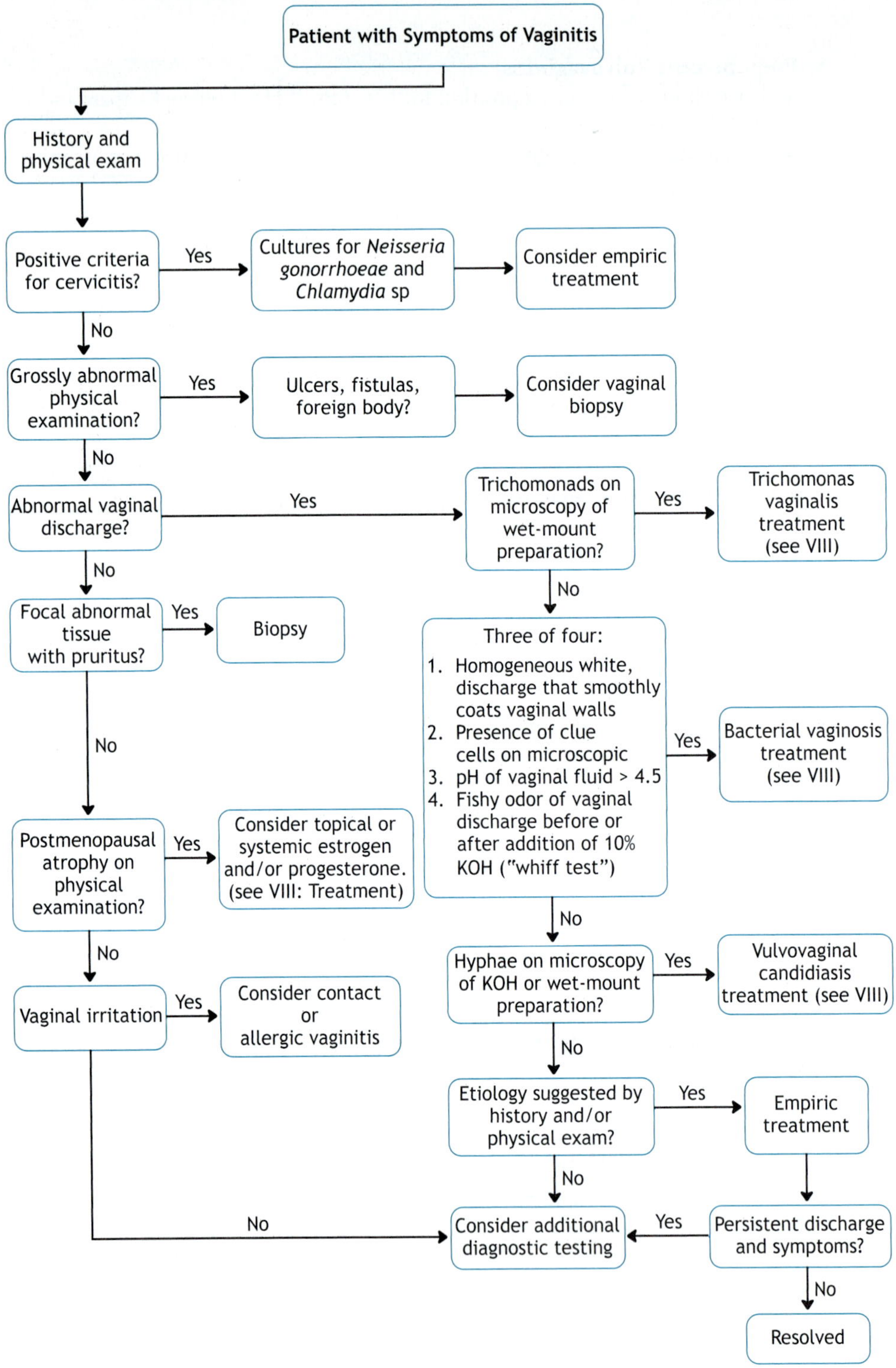

Figure 22–1. Care of the patient with symptoms of vaginitis.

d. If the uterus has not been removed, progesterone should be considered. This can be added as medroxyprogesterone (Provera) 2.5 mg daily or 10 mg for 10 days of each month.
e. Conjugated estrogen vaginal cream (2–4 g/day intravaginally)

E. **Prepubescent Vulvovaginitis**
1. **Hygiene**
a. Wipe front-to-back after elimination.
b. Avoid bubble baths and other irritating products.
c. Clean vaginal area daily with mild soap and water, drying gently with soft towel or cool hair dryer.
d. Apply bland ointments for protection of the skin, if necessary.
2. **Pharmacotherapy**
a. **Empiric treatment:** amoxicillin 20 mg/kg/day for 7 days; in areas of high prevalence of *Haemophilus influenzae*-resistant infection, use amoxicillin-clavulanate (Augmentin) 20 mg/kg/day.
b. **Estrogen deficiency with labial adhesion/agglutination:** Apply estrogen conjugated cream to fused area nightly for 2 weeks.
c. **Specific organisms on culture**
(1) **Group A β Streptococcus, *Streptococcus pneumoniae:*** Penicillin V (Pen-Vee K) 25–50 mg/kg/day, maximum of 3 gm/day, divided qid x 10 days
(2) ***H influenzae:*** Amoxicillin 20–40 mg/kg/day x 7 days; amoxicillin-clavulanate 20 mg/kg/day
(3) ***Staphylococcus aureus:*** Cephalexin 25–50 mg/kg/day, divided qid x 7–10 days or dicloxacillin 12.5–25 mg/kg/day x 7–10 days
(4) ***Candida* spp:** Topical nystatin (Mycostatin), miconazole, clotrimazole, or terconazole

IX. Summary Table

Condition	Pathophysiology	Diagnostic Studies	Treatment
Bacterial vaginosis	Replacement of normal vaginal flora	pH of vaginal discharge; "whiff test"; microscopic exam of discharge with KOH and saline solutions	Metronidazole
Candidal vaginitis	Infection with *Candida* sp.	pH of vaginal discharge; "whiff test"; microscopic exam of discharge with KOH and saline solutions	Intravaginal topical antifungal
Trichomoniasis	Infection with *T vaginalis*	pH of vaginal discharge; "whiff test"; microscopic exam of discharge with KOH and saline solutions	Metronidazole

(continued)

Summary Table (continued)

Condition	Pathophysiology	Diagnostic Studies	Treatment
Estrogen-related vulvovaginitis	Loss of estrogen	None	Estrogen (topical or intravaginal)
Contact vulvovaginitis (form of prepubescent vulvovaginitis)	Exposure to irritant	None	Avoidance of irritant

CLINICAL CASE

A 20-year-old college student presents with a complaint of a vaginal discharge. She states that the odor is "nasty" and seems to be worse after intercourse. It looks dirty-white. She states that she has had yeast infections before, but this is different because it does not itch like the yeast infections she has had. She has had 4 male sex partners since becoming sexually active 2 years ago. She recently started having relations with a new boyfriend. She takes oral contraceptive pills but does not use condoms. She says she knows her boyfriend is "safe." She says that she had a normal menstrual period 3 weeks ago. She began menstruation at age 12 and has had periods regularly every 4 weeks, and they last 4 days. She does not have excessive bleeding. Her past medical history is non-contributory, as is her family history. There is no diabetes in her family. She drinks a few beers on Friday and Saturday nights. She does not use tobacco. She "snorted" cocaine once, but currently does not use it or any other illegal drugs. She is doing "okay" in school. On physical examination, she appears healthy. Her vital signs are all normal. Her BMI is 19.3. HEENT and heart and lung examinations are normal. Vaginal examination shows no vulvar irritation, but there is a gray-white discharge in the vaginal vault. The cervical os appears non-parous, and there is no inflammation apparent. Her bimanual examination reveals a normally placed, non-gravid uterus. There is no cervical motion or adnexal tenderness. The vaginal discharge taken during the examination is placed on two slides: one with KOH solution and the other with saline solution. The KOH preparation emits a fishy odor. Microscopic examination of the KOH slide reveals no hyphae. Examination of the saline slide reveals no trichomonads. There are epithelial cells studded with bacteria along the periphery of the clue cells.

Our patient has vaginitis. The three common vaginitides are trichomonas vaginalis, bacterial vaginosis, and candidal vaginitis. It is often helpful to obtain the patient's history to differentiate among the three causes of vaginitis (see V).

Our patient has bacterial vaginosis. Although inflammatory vaginal symptoms are often absent, the foul smell is significant and may be the main reason that our patient sought medical care. Although physicians commonly confirm a diagnosis when they see clue cells (epithelial cells studded with bacteria), the **diagnostic criteria require 3 of the following 4 signs or symptoms:**

1. Homogeneous white, noninflammatory discharge that smoothly coats the vaginal walls.

2. Presence of clue cells on microscopic examination.
3. pH of vaginal fluid > 4.5.
4. Fishy odor of vaginal discharge before or after addition of 10% KOH solution (ie, the "whiff test").

A pH test of vaginal fluid is a simple test and is relatively easy to do using pH paper when performing the vaginal examination. A small piece of paper is placed in the discharge collected, and the color change is compared to the color indicator on the pH pager dispenser. This test allows us to follow guidelines for diagnosis. **Bacterial vaginosis is the most prevalent cause of vaginal discharge or malodor;** however, up to 50% of women with bacterial vaginosis may not report symptoms of bacterial vaginosis.

The established benefits of therapy for bacterial vaginosis in non-pregnant women are to relieve vaginal symptoms and signs of infection and reduce the risk of infectious complications after abortion or hysterectomy. Other potential benefits include the reduction of other infectious complications (eg, HIV and other STDs). **All women who have symptomatic disease require treatment** (see VIII).

Follow-up visits are unnecessary if symptoms resolve. Because recurrence of bacterial vaginosis is not unusual, women should be advised to return for additional therapy if symptoms recur. A different treatment regimen may be used to treat recurrent disease. No long-term maintenance regimen with any therapeutic agent is recommended. The results of clinical trials indicate that a woman's response to therapy and the likelihood of relapse or recurrence are not affected by treatment of her sex partner(s). Therefore, routine treatment of sex partners is not recommended.

Other causes of vaginitis are listed in the Summary Table. Although it was apparent from our patient's chief complaint that she had vaginitis, completing a history and physical examination helped to differentiate among the various causes.

CLINICAL PEARLS

Perform a "whiff test" on the vaginal discharge as well as a test for pH.

CHAPTER 23
WELL CHILD CARE

I. Defining Features: Ongoing care of children includes these essential components that together formulate well child care.

- **A.** Interval history taking
- **B.** Complete physical examination
- **C.** Appropriate, periodic screening tests
- **D.** Developmental assessment
- **E.** Tracking growth
- **F.** Immunizations
- **G.** Anticipatory guidance regarding child-rearing issues

II. Epidemiology

- **A.** Approximately **76.6% of children receive recommended well child care.**
- **B.** The immunization coverage of preschool-aged children ranged from 87.19% for varicella vaccine to 93.46% for hepatitis B vaccine.
- **C.** The immunization coverage for kindergarten-aged children ranged from 93.32% for varicella vaccine to 95.95% for measles-mumps-rubella (MMR) vaccine.
- **D.** The immunization coverage for first graders ranged from 94.4% for varicella vaccine to 95.37% for mumps vaccine.
- **E.** In 2003, coverage of the 4:3:1:3:3 series of immunizations ranged from 94% in Connecticut to 67.5% in Colorado. The **4:3:1:3:3 series comprises.**
  1. 4 doses of diphtheria, tetanus toxoids, and pertussis (DTP) vaccine; tetanus and diphtheria toxoids (Td); and diphtheria, tetanus toxoids, and acellular pertussis (DTP/DT/DTaP) vaccine:
  2. 3 doses of poliovirus vaccine
  3. 1 dose of measles-containing vaccine (MCV)
  4. 3 doses of *Haemophilus influenzae* type B vaccine (Hib)
  5. 3 doses of hepatitis B vaccine (hep B)
- **F.** Immunization rates for DTP, polio, Hib, hep B, and MMR ranged from 87% to 84%, with an overall coverage rate of 75%.
- **G.** The percentage of children who receive immunizations in primary care settings varied from 72% in office-based settings to 85% in staff model health maintenance organizations.

H. One fourth of the deaths of persons aged 10–24 years are homicides or suicides.

I. Approximately **61.5% of children aged 9–13 years do not participate in any organized physical activity during after-school hours.** Approximately 22.6% do not engage in any physical activity when they have unscheduled activities (free time).

III. Risk Factors

A. **Factors that reduced the likelihood of children receiving well child examinations were**

1. Children who are uninsured.
2. Children who are non-Hispanic white.
3. Children who have a parent who is not college educated.
4. Children who are in poor health.
5. Serious illness (Table 23-1)

B. **Children who did not receive recommended dental visits were more likely to be**

1. African American
2. Uninsured
3. From families with low incomes

Table 23-1. True contraindications to receiving immunizations.

True contraindications are moderate or severe illness: Moderate or severe illness is defined as:
Temperature: ≥ 38.5 °C (101.3 °F) (≥ 38.0 °C [100.4 °F] in children ≤ 3 months)
Acute respiratory illness with respiratory distress accompanied by any of the following: tachypnea, retractions, hypoxia; use of β-agonists over patient's baseline; administration of β-agonists or epinephrine in the clinic; addition of steroids to patient's regimen; or radiographic studies obtained
Possible serious bacterial illness: bacteremia, cellulitis, osteomyelitis, meningitis, pneumonia, septic arthritis, pyelonephritis, and urinary tract infections in children ≤ 2 years. Serious bacterial illness was suspected if any of the following was documented: 1. Patient descriptors such as sick, ill-appearing, toxic 2. Findings on examination consistent with serious bacterial illness, including rales and neck stiffness 3. Laboratory or radiologic studies obtained to rule out serious bacterial illness, including white blood cell counts, blood culture, urine culture, cerebrospinal fluid culture, and chest x-ray 4. Prognoses that suggested serious bacterial illness: rule out illnesses such as probable pneumonia or possible bacteremia
Transfer to emergency department or for hospitalization
Seizure: new-onset seizure, seizure within 48 hours, or increasing seizure frequency on current therapy
Serious injuries, trauma, fractures, or lacerations

4. Have a parent who is not college educated
5. Have postponed dental care in the past year.

IV. Clinical Presentation

A. Children often arrive for their well child care visits without any complaints.

B. Multiple abnormalities may be encountered during the physical examination, including heart murmurs. The physician must then understand when to investigate an asymptomatic finding.

C. Parents may have many questions about their child's growth and development and behavior.

CLINICAL SKILLS TIP

Most well child care activities, including immunizations, can be administered and addressed even if the child has an intercurrent illness (see Table 23–1).

V. Diagnostic Tests: Table 23–2 summarizes the periodicity of pediatric care and includes history and anticipatory guidance. Selected details of the table are presented below.

A. **Initial and Interval History** (always include)

1. Skin, hair, nails
2. Ears, hearing
3. Eyes, vision (red reflex)
4. Mouth, head, neck
5. Heart
6. Lungs
7. Abdomen
8. Genitourinary, extremities
9. Spine (scoliosis)
10. Neurological

B. **Anticipatory guidance is a critical part of pediatric care.** In each age group, there are common components (see Table 23–3). Additional components for specific age groupings include

1. **4 months:** Teething, choking, solid foods
2. **6 months:** Finger foods, cup use, interaction with parents, teething, teeth brushing
3. **9 months:** Mobility safety, finger foods, self-feeding, interaction with parents, wean from bottle, cup use
4. **12 months:** Sleep practice, drowning prevention, nutrition, self-feeding, wean from bottle, cup use, car seat, mobility, discipline, praise
5. **15 months:** Sleep practices, drowning prevention, nutrition, temper tantrums, interaction with parents reading, discipline, limits
6. **18 months:** Sleep practices, dental caries prevention, nutrition, mealtimes, sibling interaction, read to child, interaction with parents reading, discipline, limits
7. **24 months:** Sleep practice, car seat, dental caries prevention nutrition, exercise, toilet training, sun safety
8. **3 year old:** Toilet training, car seat, reading, preschool
9. **4 year old**: Toilet training, car seat

10. **5 years old:** Street safety, car seat, seat belts, air bags, tooth brushing twice per day, school readiness
11. **6 years old:** Sport and injury prevention, dental sealants, seat belts and air bags, street safety, age appropriate behavior, sport and bike helmet use,
12. **8 years old:** Seat belts and air bags, street safety, age appropriate behavior, sport and bike helmet use
13. **10–13 years old:** Dental care and flossing, self-care, education goals and activities, social interaction, seat belts and air bags, sex education, depression and anxiety, sports and injury prevention, self control, tobacco, alcohol, drugs, and inhalants, peer refusal skills, violence prevention, and gun safety
14. **14–21 years old:** As noted in several tables, additional items are addressed during adolescence. The mnemonic **HEADS** can be used to guide the history taking with an adolescent: **H**ome; **E**ducation and employment; **A**ctivities; **D**rugs; **S**exuality (Table 23–4).

CLINICAL CASE

A mother brings her 15-month-old child for an urgent care visit with the complaint of fever and fussiness. The mother says that the boy developed a fever of 37.9 °C (100.3 °F) the previous evening. She gave him acetaminophen, and he slept well through the night without any other problems. This morning he had a fever again and did not eat his breakfast. The mother says that he does not seem to have any abdominal complaints and is not experiencing diarrhea. She is worried that he has an infection and wants him treated with antibiotics. His past history is significant for multiple urgent care visits with diagnoses of viral illness, upper respiratory infection, and otitis media. He was delivered vaginally at term and weighed 3.4 kg (7 lb 8 oz). The mother's pregnancy was uncomplicated. The child's neonatal course was without complications. He has reached all of his developmental milestones as expected, and he has been at the 50th percentile for height and the 75th percentile for weight. He has received his first set of immunizations. A review of his chart reveals mild febrile illnesses at the times of multiple well child care visits, and a decision was made to withhold immunizations. His family history is unremarkable. He is the only child of a 22-year-old single mother who works full-time while the child is in day care. There is no exposure to secondhand smoke. On physical examination, he appears non-toxic. His temperature is 37.7 °C (99.8 °F). HEENT examination reveals normal tympanic membranes with a normal cone of light. There is no adenopathy. His chest, heart, and abdominal examinations are all normal. A urinalysis reveals a specific gravity of 1.009 and is negative for leukocytes.

As an urgent care visit, **this child may have a minor viral illness because there is no identifiable bacterial illness** (otitis media, pneumonia, gastroenteritis). The mother should be praised for treating the child with acetaminophen to help build her confidence in her ability to care for her child. As noted in Chapter 8 in the case on cough due to a viral illness, this child does not need antibiotics. However, as indicated from your review of his chart, he has received only one set of immunizations. Although the child came to see you as an urgent care visit, **he needs preventive well child care.**

Multiple studies have highlighted the missed opportunities for well child care and the inappropriate reasons to withhold immunizations. The Advisory Committee on Immunization Practices (ACIP) has issued guidelines regarding withholding immunizations and

Table 23–2. Periodicity of pediatric care.

Recommendations for Preventive Pediatric Health Care (RE9535)
Committee on Practice and Ambulatory Medicine

Each child and family is unique; therefore, these **Recommendations for Preventive Pediatric Health Care** are designed for the care of children who are receiving competent parenting, have no manifestations of any important health problems, and are growing and developing in satisfactory fashion. **Additional visits may become necessary** if circumstances suggest variations from normal.

	INFANCY[4]								
AGE[5]	**Prenatal[1]**	**Newborn[2]**	**2–4d[3]**	**By 1mo**	**2mo**	**4mo**	**6mo**	**9mo**	**12mo**
HISTORY									
Initial/Interval	•	•	•	•	•	•	•	•	•
MEASUREMENTS									
Height and Weight		•	•	•	•	•	•	•	•
Head Circumference		•	•	•	•	•	•	•	•
Blood Pressure									
SENSORY SCREENING									
Vision		S	S	S	S	S	S	S	S
Hearing		O[7]	S	S	S	S	S	S	S
DEVELOPMENTAL/ BEHAVIORAL ASSESSMENT[6]		•	•	•	•	•	•	•	•
PHYSICAL EXAMINATION[9]		•	•	•	•	•	•	•	•
PROCEDURES-GENERAL[10]									
Hereditary/Metabolic Screening		←	•	→					
Immunization		•	•	•	•	•	•	•	•
Hematocrit or Hemoglobin								•	→
Urinalysis									
PROCEDURES-PATIENTS AT RISK									
Lead Screening[16]								*	→
Tuberculin Test[17]									*
Cholesterol Screening[18]									
STD Screening[19]									
Pelvic Exam[20]									
ANTICIPATORY GUIDANCE[21]	•	•	•	•	•	•	•	•	•
Injury Prevention[22]	•	•	•	•	•	•	•	•	•
Violence prevention[23]	•	•	•	•	•	•	•	•	•
Sleep Positioning Counseling[24]	•	•	•	•	•	•	•		
Nutrition Counseling[25]	•	•	•	•	•	•	•	•	•
DENTAL REFERRAL[26]									←

These guidelines represent a consensus by the Committee on Practice and Ambulatory Medicine in consultation with national committees and sections of the American Academy of Pediatrics. The Committee emphasizes the great importance of **continuity of care** in comprehensive health supervision and the need to avoid **fragmentation of care**.

EARLY CHILDHOOD[4]					MIDDLE CHILDHOOD[4]				ADOLESCENCE[4]										
15mo	18mo	24mo	3y	4y	5y	6y	8y	10y	11y	12y	13y	14y	15y	16y	17y	18y	19y	20y	21y
•	•	•	•	•	•	•	•	•	•	•	•	•	•	•	•	•	•	•	•
•	•	•	•	•	•	•	•	•	•	•	•	•	•	•	•	•	•	•	•
•	•	•																	
			•	•	•	•	•	•	•	•	•	•	•	•	•	•	•	•	•
S	S	S	O[6]	O	O	O	O	O	S	O	S	S	O	S	S	O	S	S	S
S	S	S	S	O	O	O	O	O	S	O	S	S	O	S	S	O	S	S	S
•	•	•	•	•	•	•	•	•	•	•	•	•	•	•	•	•	•	•	•
•	•	•	•	•	•	•	•	•	•	•	•	•	•	•	•	•	•	•	•
•	•	•	•	•	•	•	•	•	•	•	•	•	•	•	•	•	•	•	•
*——	——	——	——	——	→				←——	——	•[14]	——	——	——	——	——	——	——	→
					•				←——	——	——	——	——	•[15]	——	——	——	——	→
		*																	
*	*	*	*	*	*	*	*	*	*	*	*	*	*	*	*	*	*	*	*
		*	*	*	*	*	*	*	*	*	*	*	*	*	*	*	*	*	*
									*	*	*	*	*	*	*	*	*	*	*
									*	*	*	*	*	*	*	*←	*[20]	*	→*
•	•	•	•	•	•	•	•	•	•	•	•	•	•	•	•	•	•	•	•
•	•	•	•	•	•	•	•	•	•	•	•	•	•	•	•	•	•	•	•
•	•	•	•	•	•	•	•	•	•	•	•	•	•	•	•	•	•	•	•
•	•	•	•	•	•	•	•	•	•	•	•	•	•	•	•	•	•	•	•
——	——	——	——	•															

(continued)

Table 23–2. Periodicity of pediatric care. (continued)

1. A prenatal visit is recommended for parents who are at high risk, for first-time parents, and for those who request a conference. The prenatal visit should include anticipatory guidance, pertinent medical history, and a discussion of benefits of breastfeeding and planned method of feeding per AAP statement "The Prenatal Visit" (1996).
2. Every infant should have a newborn evaluation after birth. Breastfeeding should be encouraged and instruction and support offered. Every breastfeeding infant should have an evaluation 48–72 hours after discharge from the hospital to include weight, formal breastfeeding evaluation, encouragement, and instruction as recommended in the AAP statement "Breastfeeding and the Use of Human Milk" (1997).
3. For newborns discharged in less than 48 hours after delivery per AAP statement "Hospital Stay for Healthy Term Newborns" (1995).
4. Developmental, psychosocial, and chronic disease issues for children and adolescents may require frequent counseling and treatment visits separate from preventive care visits.
5. If a child comes under care for the first time at any point on the schedule, or if any items are not accomplished at the suggested age, the schedule should be brought up to date at the earliest possible time.
6. If the patient is uncooperative, rescreen within 6 months.
7. All newborns should be screened per the AAP Task Force on Newborn and Infant Hearing statement, "Newborn and Infant Hearing Loss: Detection and Intervention" (1999).
8. By history and appropriate physical examination: if suspicious, by specific objective developmental testing. Parenting skills should be fostered at every visit.
9. At each visit, a complete physical examination is essential, with infant totally unclothed, older child undressed and suitably draped.
10. These may be modified, depending upon entry point into schedule and individual need.
11. Metabolic screening (eg, thyroid, hemoglobinopathies, PKU, galactosemia) should be done according to state law.
12. Schedule(s) per the Committee on Infectious Diseases, published annually in the January edition of *Pediatrics*. Every visit should be an opportunity to update and complete a child's immunizations.
13. See AAP *Pediatric Nutrition Handbook* (1998) for a discussion of universal and selective screening options. Consider earlier screening for high-risk infants (eg, premature infants and low birth weight infants). See also "Recommendations to Prevent and Control Iron Deficiency in the United States. *MMWR*. 1998;47 (RR-3):1-29.

Key: • = to be performed; * = to be performed for patients at risk
S = subjective, by history; O = objective, by a standard testing method
◄—•—► = the range during which a service may be provided, with the dot indicating the preferred age.

14. All menstruating adolescents should be screened annually.
15. Conduct dipstick urinalysis for leukocytes annually for sexually active male and female adolescents.
16. For children at risk of lead exposure consult the AAP statement "Screening for Elevated Blood Levels" (1998). Additionally, screening should be done in accordance with state law where applicable.
17. TB testing per recommendations of the Committee on Infectious Diseases, published in the current edition of *Red Book: Report of the Committee on Infectious Diseases.* Testing should be done upon recognition of high-risk factors.
18. Cholesterol screening for high-risk patients per AAP statement "Cholesterol in Childhood" (1998). If family history cannot be ascertained and other risk factors are present, screening should be at the discretion of the physician.
19. All sexually active patients should be screened for sexually transmitted diseases (STDs).
20. All sexually active females should have a pelvic examination. A pelvic examination and routine pap smear should be offered as part of preventive health maintenance between the ages of 18 and 21 years.
21. Age-appropriate discussion and counseling should be an integral part of each visit for care per the AAP *Guidelines for Health Supervision III* (1998).
22. From birth to age 12, refer to the AAP injury prevention program (TIPP®) as described in *A Guide to Safety Counseling in Office Practice* (1994).
23. Violence prevention and management for all patients per AAP Statement "The Role of the Pediatrician in Youth Violence Prevention in Clinical Practice and at the Community Level" (1999).
24. Parents and caregivers should be advised to place healthy infants on their backs when putting them to sleep. Side positioning is a reasonable alternative but carries a slightly higher risk of SIDS. Consult the AAP statement "Positioning and Sudden Infant Death Syndrome (SIDS): Update" (1996).
25. Age-appropriate nutrition counseling should be an integral part of each visit per the AAP *Handbook of Nutrition* (1998).
26. Earlier initial dental examinations may be appropriate for some children. Subsequent examinations as prescribed by dentist.

NB: Special chemical, immunologic, and endocrine testing is usually carried out upon specific indications. Testing other than newborn (eg, inborn errors of metabolism, sickle disease, etc) is discretionary with the physician.

The recommendations in this statement do not indicate an exclusive course of treatment or standard of medical care. Variations taking into account individual circumstances, may be appropriate.

From: The American Academy of Pediatrics.

Table 23–3. Anticipatory guidance by age group.

Age Group	Common Elements of Anticipatory Guidance
Birth–24 months	• Supine sleep position • Drowning prevention • Postpartum adjustment • Dental gum care • Signs of illness • Passive smoke • Family involvement • Injury prevention • Car seat • Infant bonding • Emergency and 911 • Parenting practices • Next appointment and transportation needed
Aged 3–13 years	• Drowning prevention • Sport helmet use • Passive smoke • Social interaction • Sun safety • Nutrition/exercise • Reading • Family involvement • Dental caries prevention • Discipline • "Safe at home?" • Next appointment and transportation needed
Aged 13–21 years	• Drowning and sun safety • Education goals and activities • Dental and self care • Social interaction • "Safe at home?" • Seat belts and driving safety • Sex education/counseling • Depression and anxiety • Parenting advice • Sports and injury prevention • Self control • Tobacco, alcohol, drugs, inhalants • Family involvement • Nutrition/exercise • Peer refusal skills • Violence prevention and gun safety • Next appointment.

Table 23–4. HEADS: Examples of good and bad opening lines.

	BAD	GOOD	REASON WHY
Home	Tell me about Mom & Dad	Where do you live and who lives there with you?	Parent(s) may have died or left home. Open-ended questions enable the physician to collect "environmental" as well as personal history.
Education	How are you doing in school?	What are you good at in school? What is hard for you? What grades do you get?	Poor questions can be "OK." Good questions ask for information about strengths and weaknesses and allow for quantification.
Activities	Do you have any activities outside of school?	What do you do for fun? What things do you do with your friends? What do you do when you have free time?	Good questions are open-ended and allow a patient to express him/herself.
Drugs	Do you do drugs?	Many young people experiment with drugs, alcohol, or cigarettes. Have you or your friends ever tried them?	Good question is an expression of concern with follow-up. With younger teenagers it is best to begin by asking about friends.
Sexuality	Have you ever had sex? Tell me about your boy/girl friend.	Have you ever had a sexual relationship with anyone? Most people become interested in sexual relationships at your age. Have you had any with boys, girls, or both? Tell me about your sex life.	What does the term "have sex" really mean to teenagers? Asking only about heterosexual relationships closes doors at once.

regards minor illnesses as an inappropriate reason to withhold immunizations. The expectation that the child will return within a few days when the illness is resolved is not an appropriate course of action.

In one of many studies examining missed opportunities for immunization administration, it was found that these opportunities occurred in 47% of the appropriate occasions to administer the vaccines. Only 40% of the children with missed opportunities for immunization received age-appropriate immunizations within 6 months; 30% received the vaccinations beyond the age-appropriate time. The remaining 30% either did not return or were not vaccinated on return. The variables significantly associated with missed opportunities were listed as age: children with missed opportunities were older than those without a missed opportunity, with a mean age of 15.5 months vs 10.9 months; minor febrile illness; moderate/severe illness; acute illness encounters; and the patient was being seen at the community health center. Only 15.5% of all missed opportunities were justified by the presence of moderate to severe illness.

Table 23–5. Childhood immunization schedule.

Department of Health and Human Services • Centers for Disease Control and Prevention

Recommended Childhood and Adolescent Immunization Schedule UNITED STATES • 2006

Vaccine ▼ / Age ▶	Birth	1 month	2 months	4 months	6 months	12 months	15 months	18 months	24 months	4–6 years	11–12 years	13–14 years	15 years	16–18 years
Hepatitis B[1]	HepB	HepB		*HepB[1]*		HepB						HepB Series		
Diphtheria, Tetanus, Pertussis[2]			DTaP	DTaP	DTaP		DTaP			DTaP	Tdap		Tdap	
Haemophilus influenzae type b[3]			Hib	Hib	*Hib[3]*	Hib								
Inactivated Poliovirus			IPV	IPV		IPV				IPV				
Measles, Mumps, Rubella[4]						MMR				MMR		MMR		
Varicella[5]							Varicella				Varicella			
Meningococcal[6]								Vaccines within broken line are for selected populations	MPSV4		MCV4		MCV4 MCV4	
Pneumococcal[7]			PCV	PCV	PCV	PCV			PCV		PPV			
Influenza[8]						Influenza (Yearly)					Influenza (Yearly)			
Hepatitis A[9]										HepA Series				

This schedule indicates the recommended ages for routine administration of currently licensed childhood vaccines, as of December 1, 2005, for children through age 18 years. Any dose not administered at the recommended age should be administered at any subsequent visit when indicated and feasible. ▒ Indicates age groups that warrant special effort to administer those vaccines not previously administered. Additional vaccines may be licensed and recommended during the year. Licensed combination vaccines may be used whenever any components of the combination are indicated and other components of the vaccine are not contraindicated and if approved by the Food and Drug Administration for that dose of the series. Providers should consult the respective ACIP statement for detailed recommendations. Clinically significant adverse events that follow immunization should be reported to the Vaccine Adverse Event Reporting System (VAERS). Guidance about how to obtain and complete a VAERS form is available at **www.vaers.hhs.gov** or by telephone, 800-822-7967.

▒ Range of recommended ages ▒ Catch-up immunization ▒ 11–12 year old assessment

1. **Hepatitis B vaccine (HepB).** ***AT BIRTH:*** **All newborns** should receive monovalent HepB soon after birth and before hospital discharge. **Infants born to mothers who are HBsAg-positive** should receive HepB and 0.5 mL of hepatitis B immune globulin (HBIG) within 12 hours of birth. **Infants born to mothers whose HBsAg status is unknown** should receive HepB within 12 hours of birth. The mother should have blood drawn as soon as possible to determine her HBsAg status; if HBsAg-positive, the infant should receive HBIG as soon as possible (no later than age 1 week). **For infants born to HBsAg-negative mothers,** the birth dose can be delayed in rare circumstances but only if a physician's order to withhold the vaccine and a copy of the mother's original HBsAg-negative laboratory report are documented in the infant's medical record. ***FOLLOWING THE BIRTH-DOSE:*** The HepB series should be completed with either monovalent HepB or a combination vaccine containing HepB. The second dose should be administered at age 1–2 months. The final dose should be administered at age ≥ 24 weeks. It is permissible to administer 4 doses of HepB (e.g., when combination vaccines are given after the birth dose); however, if monovalent HepB is used, a dose at age 4 months is not needed. **Infants born to HBsAg-positive mothers** should be tested for HBsAg and antibody to HBsAg after completion of the HepB series, at age 9–18 months (generally at the next well-child visit after completion of the vaccine series).
2. **Diphtheria and tetanus toxoids and acellular pertussis vaccine (DTaP).** The fourth dose of DTaP may be administered as early as age 12 months, provided 6 months have elapsed since the third dose and the child is unlikely to return at age 15–18 months. The final dose in the series should be given at age ≥ 4 years. **Tetanus and diphtheria toxoids and acellular pertussis vaccine (Tdap-adolescent preparation)** is recommended at age 11–12 years for those who have completed the recommended childhood DTP/DTaP vaccination series and have not received a Td booster dose. Adolescents 13–18 years who missed the 11–12 year Td/Tdap booster dose should also receive a single dose of Tdap if they have completed the recommended childhood DTP/DTaP vaccination series. Subsequent **tetanus and diphtheria toxoids (Td)** are recommended every 10 years.
3. ***Haemophilus influenzae*** **type b conjugate vaccine (Hib).** Three Hib conjugate vaccines are licensed for infant use. If PRP-OMP (PedvaxHIB® or ComVax® [Merck]) is administered at ages 2 and 4 months, a dose at age 6 months is not required. DTaP/Hib combination products should not be used for primary immunization in infants at ages 2, 4 or 6 months but can be used as boosters after any Hib vaccine. The final dose in the series should be administered at age ≥ 12 months.
4. **Measles, mumps, and rubella vaccine (MMR).** The second dose of MMR is recommended routinely at age 4–6 years but may be administered during any visit, provided at least 4 weeks have elapsed since the first dose and both doses are administered beginning at or after age 12 months. Those who have not previously received the second dose should complete the schedule by age 11–12 years.
5. **Varicella vaccine.** Varicella vaccine is recommended at any visit at or after age 12 months for susceptible children (i.e., those who lack a reliably history of chickenpox). Susceptible persons aged ≥ 13 years should receive 2 doses administered at least 4 weeks apart.
6. **Meningococcal vaccine (MCV4).** Meningococcal conjugate vaccine (MCV4) should be given to all children at the 11–12 year old visit as well as to unvaccinated adolescents at high school entry (15 years of age). Other adolescents who wish to decrease their risk for meningococcal disease may also be vaccinated. All college freshmen living in dormitories should be vaccinated, preferably with MCV4, although **meningococcal polysaccharide vaccine (MPSV4)** is an acceptable alternative. Vaccination against invasive meningococcal disease is recommended for children and adolescents aged ≥ 2 years with terminal complement deficiencies or anatomic or functional asplenia and certain other high risk groups (see *MMWR* 2005;54 [RR-7]:1-21); use MPSV4 for children aged 2–10 years and MCV4 for older children, although MPSV4 is an acceptable alternative.
7. **Pneumococcal vaccine.** The heptavalent **pneumococcal conjugate vaccine (PCV)** is recommended for all children aged 2–23 months and for certain children aged 24–59 months. The final dose in the series should be given at age ≥ 12 months. **Pneumococcal polysaccharide vaccine (PPV)** is recommended in addition to PCV for certain high-risk groups. See *MMWR* 2000;49(RR-9):1-35.

(*continued*)

Table 23–5. Childhood immunization schedule. (continued)

8. **Influenza vaccine.** Influenza vaccine is recommended annually for children aged ≥ 6 months with certain risk factors (including, but not limited to, asthma, cardiac disease, sickle cell disease, human immunodeficiency virus [HIV], diabetes, and conditions that can compromise respiratory function or handling of respiratory secretions or that can increase the risk for aspiration), healthcare workers, and other persons (including household members) in close contact with persons in groups at high risk (see *MMWR* 2005;54[RR-8]:1-55). In addition, healthy children aged 6–23 months and close contacts of healthy children aged 0–5 months are recommended to receive influenza vaccine because children in this age group are at substantially increased risk for influenza-related hospitalizations. For healthy persons aged 5–49 years, the intranasally administered, live, attenuated influenza vaccine (LAIV) is an acceptable alternative to the intramuscular trivalent inactivated influenza vaccine (TIV). See *MMWR* 2005;54(RR-8):1-55. Children receiving TIV should be administered a dosage appropriate for their age (0.25 mL if aged 6–35 months or 0.5 mL if aged ≥ 3 years). Children aged ≤ 8 years who are receiving influenza vaccine for the first time should receive 2 doses (separated by at least 4 weeks for TIV and at least 6 weeks for LAIV).
9. **Hepatitis A vaccine (HepA).** HepA is recommended for all children at 1 year of age (i.e., 12–23 months). The 2 doses in the series should be administered at least 6 months apart. States, counties, and communities with existing HepA vaccination programs for children 2–18 years of age are encouraged to maintain these programs. In these areas, new effort focused on routine vaccination of 1-year-old children should enhance, not replace, ongoing programs directed at a broader population of children. HepA is also recommended for certain high risk groups (see *MMWR* 1999;48[RR-12]1-37).

The Childhood and Adolescent Immunization Schedule is approved by:
Advisory Committee on Immunization Practices **www.cdc.gov/nip/acip** • American Academy of Pediatrics **www.aap.org** • American Academy of Family Physicians **ww.aafp.org**

The ACIP has defined true contraindications to receive immunizations as moderate or severe illness (see Table 23–1). Patients with moderate or severe illnesses, with or without fever, can be vaccinated as soon as they are beginning to recover and are no longer acutely ill. In the absence of a moderate or severe illness, this child should have his second set of immunizations administered as indicated in Table 23–5.

Well child care includes multiple components, in addition to immunizations, depending on the child's age (see V).

Although many health plans have specific forms to be completed at each well child visit, such as the Early Periodic Screening and Diagnostic Tests (EPSDT) for Medicaid patients, physicians should

1. When possible, incorporate assessments of preventive service needs and counseling and education as appropriate into acute visits.
2. Consider all clinic visits, whether acute or chronic, as opportunities to provide preventive counseling and anticipatory guidance for pediatric patients.

Counseling and anticipatory guidance are critically important aspects of well child care. Many topics are included in the lists for providers to discuss with parents; however, not all are supported by the literature (Tables 23–6, 23–7, 22–8, 23–9).

CLINICAL PEARLS

Do not miss any opportunities to provide well child care and immunizations.

Table 23–6. Topics for physician-parent discussions about children from birth to 2 years.

There is *good* evidence to support counseling on these topics. Counseling should be included in a periodic health examination.	There is *fair* evidence to support counseling on these topics. Counseling should be included in a periodic health examination.	There may be *insufficient* direct evidence that counseling on these topics leads to a specific change of behavior; however, there is evidence linking these topics to health conditions and/or diseases.
• Breast feeding • Viral upper respiratory infection	• Iron rich diet • Physical activity • Child safety seats • Poison prevention • Flame-resistant sleepwear • Protection from ultraviolet (UV) light • Infant sleep position and sudden infant death syndrome (SIDS) • Dental and periodontal disease • Infants and bottles	• Formula use • Motor vehicles, bicycles • Safety helmets • Fire safety • Poison, water safety, and choking • Falls • Water heater safety • Firearm storage • Promotion of nonviolent behavior and screen for family violence • Coping skills and stress reduction • Preventive care visits • Fluoride supplements

Table 23–7. Topics for physician-parent discussions about children aged 2–6 years.

There is *good* evidence to support counseling on these topics. Counseling should be included in a periodic health examination.	There is *fair* evidence to support counseling on these topics. Counseling should be included in a periodic health examination.	There may be *insufficient* direct evidence that counseling on these topics leads to a specific change of behavior; however, there is evidence linking these topics to health conditions and/or diseases.
	• Iron rich diet • Physical activity • Child safety seats • Poison prevention • Flame-resistant sleepwear • Safety belts • Protection from ultraviolet (UV) light • Dental and periodontal disease	• 5 servings per day (fruits and vegetables) • Parent role models • Healthy snacks • Calcium intake • Motor vehicles and bicycles • Safety helmets • Fire safety • Poison, water safety, and choking • Falls • Water heater safety • Firearm storage • Promotion of nonviolent behavior and screen for family violence • Coping skills/stress reduction • Preventive care visits • Fluoride supplements

Table 23–8. Topics for physician-parent discussions about children aged 7–12 years.

There is *good* evidence to support counseling on these topics. Counseling should be included in a periodic health examination.	There is *fair* evidence to support counseling on these topics. Counseling should be included in a periodic health examination.	There may be *insufficient* direct evidence that counseling on these topics leads to a specific change of behavior; however, there is evidence linking these topics to health conditions and/or diseases.
• Limited saturated fat	• Caloric balance/nutrient balance • Physical activity • Poison prevention • Flame-resistant sleepwear • Safety belts • Protection from ultraviolet (UV) light • Dental and periodontal disease	• 5 servings per day (fruits and vegetables) • Parent role models • Healthy snacks • Calcium intake • Motor vehicles, bicycles • Safety helmets • Fire safety • Poison, water safety, and choking • Firearm storage • Promotion of nonviolent behavior and screen for family violence • Coping skills and stress reduction • Preventive care visits • Fluoride supplements

Table 23–9. Topics for physician-parent discussions about children aged 13–18 years.

There is *good* evidence to support counseling on these topics. Counseling should be included in a periodic health examination.	There is *fair* evidence to support counseling on these topics. Counseling should be included in a periodic health examination.	There may be *insufficient* direct evidence that counseling on these topics leads to a specific change of behavior; however, there is evidence linking these topics to health conditions and/or diseases.
• Limited saturated fat • Folic acid supplements • Tobacco cessation • Problem drinking	• Caloric balance/nutrient balance • Physical activity • Drinking and driving motor vehicles • Safety belts • Unintended pregnancy prevention • Protection from ultraviolet (UV) light • Dental and periodontal disease	• 5 servings per day (fruits and vegetables) • Parent role models • Healthy snacks • Calcium intake • Start of tobacco use • Alcohol and other drugs • Motor vehicle operation • Motor vehicles, bicycles • Helmets for motorcyclists • Safety helmets • Fire safety • Firearm storage • Promotion of nonviolent behavior and screen for family violence • Sexually transmitted disease prevention • Depression and anxiety awareness • Coping skills and stress reduction • Preventive care visits • Preconception counseling

APPENDIX
USEFUL WEB SITES

Allergic Rhinitis
http://www.cdc.gov/ncidod/dbmd/antibioticresistance/files/Rhinipac.pdf

Asthma
http://www.nhlbi.nih.gov/health/public/lung/asthma/asthma.htm#plan

Contraception
http://www.who.int/reproductive-health/pages_resources/listing_family_planning.htm

Cough
http://www.cdc.gov/drugresistance/community//files/ads/Practpac.pdf
http://www.cdc.gov/drugresistance/community//files/A_New_Threat_to_Your_Health.pdf

Hypercholesterolemia
http://www.nhlbi.nih.gov/guidelines/cholesterol/

Hypertension
http://www.nhlbi.nih.gov/guidelines/hypertension/

Osteoarthritis
http://www.aaos.org

Well Child Care
http://www.mchb.hrsa.gov/chusa03/pages/intro.htm

INDEX

Note: Page numbers followed by *t* and *f* indicate tables and figures, respectively.